Nursing Centers: Meeting the Demand for Quality Health Care

Pub. No. 21-2311

National League for Nursing • New York

Copyright © 1989 by
National League for Nursing

ISBN 0-88737-472-7

Manufactured in the United States of America

Contents

Contributors

Esther L. Acree, MSN, SpClNsg, FNP
Assistant Professor/Coordinator, Sycamore Nursing Center,
Academic Nurse-Managed Center
Indiana State University
School of Nursing
Terre Haute, IN

Sara Jane H. Anderson, MSN, ANP, RN
Assistant Professor
College of Nursing
University of New Mexico
Geriatric Nursing Specialist
Geriatric Education and Health Management Clinics
Albuquerque, NM

Myrtle K. Aydelotte, PhD, FAAN
Professor and Dean Emeritus
College of Nursing
University of Iowa
Iowa City, IA

Sara E. Barger, DPA, RN, FAAN
Head, Department of Professional Development and Services
Associate Professor
Clemson University College of Nursing
Clemson, SC

Ellamae Branstetter, PhD, RN
Professor
College of Nursing
Arizona State University
Tempe, AZ

William C. Bridges, Jr., PhD
Associate Professor, Experimental Statistics
Clemson University College of Agricultural Sciences
Clemson, SC

Jo A. Brooks, DNS, RN, C
Assistant Head for Instructional Administration
Associate Professor and Director
Nursing Center for Family Health
School of Nursing
Purdue University
West Lafayette, IN

Norman D. Brown, EdD, MS, RN
Associate Professor
School of Nursing
University of Arkansas for Medical Sciences
at Little Rock
Little Rock, AR

Marjorie Buchanan, MS, RN
Assistant Professor/Project Director
Thomas Jefferson University
Philadelphia, PA

Richard J. Fehring, DNSc, RN
Associate Professor
Marquette University
College of Nursing
Milwaukee, WI

Paul Femea, DNSc, RN
University of Texas
Health Sciences Center at Houston
School of Nursing
Houston, TX

Marilyn Frenn, MSN, RN
Assistant Professor
Marquette University
College of Nursing
Milwaukee, WI

Patricia L. Gerrity, PhD, RN
Associate Professor/Project Director
La Salle University
Philadelphia, PA

Laurie K. Glass, PhD, RN, FAAN
Associate Professor
Director, Historical Gallery
School of Nursing
University of Wisconsin—Milwaukee
Milwaukee, WI

Melissa S. Gregory, MA, RN
Private Practitioner
Rochester, MN

Veda J. Gregory, MSN, SpClNsg, FNP
Assistant Professor/Director, Sycamore Nursing Center,
Academic Nurse-Managed Center
Indiana State University
School of Nursing
Terre Haute, IN

Zana Rae Higgs, EdD, RN
Professor, Graduate Faculty
Intercollegiate Center for Nursing Education
Spokane, WA

Elizabeth Holman, MS, RN
Adjunct Faculty and Coordinator
Community Health Services Clinic
College of Nursing
Arizona State University
Tempe, AZ

Sally Peck Lundeen, PhD, RN
Director, Nursing Center
University of Wisconsin—Milwaukee
Milwaukee, WI

Mary Ann McDermott, EdD, RN
Associate Professor
Niehoff School of Nursing
Loyola University of Chicago
Chicago, IL

Mary J. Roehrig, MSN, MA, RN
Coordinator, Nursing Center
Assistant Professor
Ferris State University
Department of Nursing
Big Rapids, MI

Preface

The turn of this century saw the birth of nursing centers across the country to help deal with the burdensome conditions of disease, poverty, and homelessness. Today, as yesterday, despite the technological and social advances we have seen, such conditions remain as a grim reminder of progress yet to be made. The nature of nursing centers, or NMCs, is such that the socioeconomic and psychosocial conditions of both society at large as well as the patients served are an integral part of what NMCs are and what they do. It is their niche, the importance of which cannot be underestimated.

It is in this spirit that we present *Nursing Centers: Meeting the Demand for Quality Health Care*, a collection of papers which were presented at the Fourth National Conference on Nursing Centers in Milwaukee, Wisconsin in May 1988. The authors explore a wide span of topics on nursing centers—from their historical conception to their daily "nuts and bolts" activity.

As we approach the next century, it is clear that many of society's problems remain unsolved, however, they are surmountable. Through hard work and a clear understanding of how society affects and is affected by these conditions, we can make a difference. It is this ethic that has inspired and guided nursing centers to make their indelible mark on today's health care scene.

Nursing Practice: Innovative Models

Myrtle K. Aydelotte, PhD, FAAN
Melissa S. Gregory, MA, RN

There is little debate that in the future the demand for nursing services and health care will be unprecedented in the amount and kinds of services needed to serve the public. The problem confronting society revolves around how nursing services will meet this demand, how they will be organized, how they will be financed, and how nurses will be educated. To address the problem, society, nurses, and the nursing profession must examine each issue associated with the problem and make choices wisely. The concept of nursing centers and innovative private-practice models holds promise in resolving the problem.

HISTORICAL PERSPECTIVE

Nursing centers in the United States, operated by nurses who wish to promote health and provide nursing care, have a long and rich history. Since the late 1800s, visiting nurses' associations have promoted health, and provided home care and health teaching to the sick and impoverished in cities throughout the United States, opening the way for the development of subsequent nursing centers. The following brief review summarizes and highlights major contributions made by various nurse leaders and organizations.[1]

---

[1]For more historical information, the reader is referred to ANA's (1987) publication, *The Nursing Center: Concept and Design.*

Lillian Wald founded the Henry Street Nurses Settlement in New York City in 1893. The nurses at this center were not only concerned with providing nursing care to the sick and impoverished, but were also actively involved with issues related to the causes of illness and health promotion.

Margaret Sanger opened the first U.S. birth control clinic in 1916. The center's goal was to provide the poor with information on contraception and family planning. Ms. Sanger became a national advocate for women's health and was politically active in the birth control movement (Douglas, 1970).

Mary Breckinridge, a certified nurse-midwife, established the Frontier Nursing Service in the remote mountains of eastern Kentucky in the 1920s. This service provided direct nursing care to mothers and babies (Breckinridge, 1981).

The Cleveland Nursing Center was established in 1920 in response to a request made by the Council of National Defense. Its purpose was to centralize nursing services and to provide a more efficient means of responding to disasters (Hodgins & Smith, 1925).

In 1963, Lydia Hall established the Loeb Center at Montefiore Hospital in New York City, to provide an institutional service "midway between hospital and home." The 80-bed facility provided intensive nursing and restorative care for patients during recovery following medical and surgical hospital care. The organization of services at Loeb Center resembled public health nursing within an institutional setting, and professional nurses were the only individuals who provided nursing care (Hall, 1963).

In 1965, the nurse practitioner role was established allowing the nurse to "provide primary care as the client's first contact in illness-related care . . . with continued responsibility for the client's health, maintenance, evaluation, and appropriate referral" (American Nurses' Association, 1987, p. 3).

In 1971, M. Lucille Kinlein established her practice to gain complete control over her actions in achieving her nursing goals. She stated, "I became convinced that the only way to identify precisely and meet satisfactorily the nursing needs of people was to change the setting in which I came into contact with persons in the need of nursing care" (Kinlein, 1972, p. 23). Kinlein described the process of meeting the client's nursing needs as providing direct physical and psychological care, emotional support, and health counseling, in states of illness and health.

The 1970s marked the beginning of many university- or academic-based nursing centers which were established to provide community services, learning sites for student experiences, a setting for faculty practice, and a setting for faculty and student research (Culbert-Hinthorn et al., 1985; (Lang, 1983). In 1987, O. Marie Henry addressed the American Public Health Association and urged nurses to develop new means for providing nursing care and delivering nursing services. She asserted that nursing centers should be established in institutional, community- and primary-care settings to provide direct access to nursing care, to promote student learning, and to foster research. Henry proposed that nursing centers be administered and coordinated by professional nurses, and that the main focus of such centers be nursing (Henry, 1978; American Nurses' Association, 1987).

The 1980s have seen a proliferation of many types of nursing centers, including academic-based, hospital-based and freestanding centers, and nurse-managed agencies for home health care. Current estimates suggest that approximately 150 academic nursing centers are now in existence in the United States, and a survey is presently underway to ascertain the number of freestanding centers (Riesch, 1987).

Nurse leaders who have been involved in the many aspects of nursing centers collectively met at the First National Conference on Nursing Centers in Milwaukee in May 1982. The meeting focused on the past, present, and future of nursing centers (Lang, 1983). At the Second National Conference, held in Milwaukee in 1984, a working definition of a nursing center was obtained through consensus of the participants via the Delphi survey method conducted by Fehring, Schulte, and Riesch (1986). The results of the survey guided the investigators in proposing the following definition of a nursing center:

> Nurse-Managed Centers are organizations that provide direct access to professional nurses who offer holistic, client-centered health services for reimbursement. With the use of nursing models of health, professional nurses in NMCs diagnose and treat human responses to potential and actual health problems. Examples of professional nursing services include health education, health promotion, and health-related research. Services are targeted to underserved individuals and groups. An effective referral system and collaboration with other health care professionals are an integral part of NMCs. As models of professional nursing practice and research, NMCs are ideal sites for faculty and student practice. They are administered by a professional nurse (Fehring, Schulte, & Riesch, 1986, p. 63).

The Third National Conference was held in Scottsdale, Arizona, in 1986, and participants identified the need to establish a national organization. Subsequently, representatives from nursing centers met in Chicago in 1987 to discuss national organization planning and development (American Nurses' Association, 1987). A task force, named by the American Nurses' Association, met prior to that meeting to develop guidelines for the establishment of nursing centers (ANA, 1987).

In summary, many individuals and organizations have impacted positively the development of nursing centers. Through continued individual and collective efforts, nursing centers may continue to thrive and provide a means for nurses to meet consumer health care needs through the delivery of nursing care and to exercise control over the nursing practice domain.

DEVELOPMENT OF PRIVATE PRACTICE IN NURSING

The 1970s and 1980s also saw marked growth in private practice or independent practice of nurses. Although private-duty nursing existed prior to the 1970s and experienced rapid growth just before the Great Depression, the renaissance of private practice in nursing in the 1970s took a form different from its earlier predecessor, resembling in large part that of the nursing center.

Private-practice nursing developed as a result of significant changes in the nursing field. The programs of education that prepared clinical nurse specialists and nurse practitioners were major forces in the development. Currently, 1,298 nurses have been identified as engaged in private or independent practice. These are individuals who own a practice and are legally liable for it.

The characteristics of private or independent practice are defined as follows:

- Nurses are the owners or proprietors of the enterprise that provides the services to clients and patients. They are financially and legally responsible for all aspects of the entity.

- Nurses define and control the nature of the services that are provided by the enterprise. Thus, nurses possess the autonomy of the practice itself.

- Nurses determine the nature of the client/patient relationship and are fully accountable for the quality of that relationship and the actions that take place in the relationship. (Aydelotte, Hardy, & Hope, 1988).

A study of 365 nurses in private practice that has just been completed (Aydelotte, Hardy, & Hope, 1988)[2] provides data for making comparisons between nursing centers and private practices in nursing. Comparisons of special interest are those relating to purpose, structure, and control. These comparisons are only roughly drawn, but a data base has been compiled that lends itself to future research.

PURPOSES OF NURSING CENTERS AND PRIVATE PRACTICES IN NURSING

The purposes of nursing centers and private-practice enterprises are alike in many respects, but different in others.

---

[2]The primary author uses the term *private practice* rather than "independent practice" since the former term is commonly used in the other professions.

The purpose of a nursing center reflects its philosophy, values, and beliefs, and those served by the profession. The purpose defines the major goals of the center. It provides a framework upon which the organizational structure of the center is built, and it limits the range of services and the clientele served (American Nurses' Association, 1987).

In reviewing the literature, it is evident that nursing centers exist for a variety of purposes. However, some common themes emerge. Academic nursing centers usually exist for the following purposes:

1. To provide an opportunity for faculty practice
2. To provide a setting in which students and faculty are able to conduct research and test nursing theories and models of practice
3. To provide learning opportunities for students
4. To provide nursing services to the community (Arlton & Miercort, 1980; Baird & Benner, 1985; Bagwell, 1987; Barger, 1986; Culbert-Hinthorn et al., 1985; Duffy & Halloran, 1986; Hauf, 1977; Mezey & Chiamulera, 1980; Ossler et al., 1982; Riesch et al., 1980)

Although a few of the academic nursing centers expressed a purpose that focused primarily on student learning, as compared to providing health care services to clients, most identified a multifold purpose that included the major themes listed.

The majority of the community-based, institutional-based, and freestanding nursing centers described a purpose that focused on the client being served and the type of nursing care practiced. The purposes of these centers include the following:

1. To promote health and prevent disease for a given target population
2. To provide direct access to professional nurses for consumers
3. To provide care consistent with the management of acute and chronic illnesses
4. To provide support services to clients and their families (Hall, 1963; Jones, 1976; Lamper-Linden, Goetz-Kular, & Wahlquist, 1984)

In general, nursing centers have been developed to provide accessible settings for faculty and students to practice nursing that is not usually administered in traditional health care settings (Fehring, Schulte, & Riesch, 1986). Most nursing centers exist for the purposes of promoting health and preventing illness; providing direct access to professional nurses for consumers, practice sites for faculty, and a setting in which research can be generated; and promoting student learning. The purpose statement reflected a client focus, a practice focus, an academic focus, or some combination of all of these. The purpose provided a framework on which the center's conceptual and organizational frameworks were developed. Thus, the purpose determined what type of nursing care is provided and to whom the care is directed.

The purposes of a private practice can only be inferred from the responses to the questionnaire. The primary reason for starting the venture was identified by the majority of the respondents as "the wish to be independent." The second reason, and that given as primary by the highly successful nurses, was the fact that "an opportunity presented itself." The two types of services provided by the nurse in private practice were services to clients and services to institutions or to professionals. The clientele they served included both urban and rural populations, the majority of whom had annual incomes over $20,000. An opportunity was provided for the respondents to indicate other services, and of those who used the opportunity, no response indicated education of students and the conduct of research. One must conclude that the purposes of private practice are to provide services to clients and to earn an income.

The review of the literature related to nursing centers and analysis of the data from the study of private practice suggest comparisons (Table 1). All three have a client focus, but they differ in research, faculty, student, and income focus.

PROVISION OF SERVICES TO CLIENTS

The services provided by a nursing center are based on the center's goals and purpose. The services reflect the needs and characteristics of the target population, as well as the skills, interests, and available resources of those providing the nursing care. Though specific services vary among different nursing centers, generally they can be categorized as (1) primary prevention and health-maintenance services, (2) direct-care services for acute and chronic conditions, and (3) comprehensive health care services that treat actual and potential health problems at all points on the health-illness continuum. Services may be narrow in scope and directed toward a very specific population, or aimed at a heterogeneous group in which case services encompass a wide range of activities. The literature describes the services that are provided by a variety of nursing centers currently operating.

The Nursing Center, located at the University of Wisconsin in Milwaukee, is an academic nursing center that provides health screening, health assessment, and information and support activities. Specific activities include (1) blood pressure, scoliosis and vision screening; (2) developmental and health assessments for preschool children and physical assessments for teenage

Table 1
Analysis of Purposes of Nursing Centers and
Private-Practice Arrangements

Type of Arrangement	Academic Center	Community Nursing Center	Private Practice
Opportunity for faculty practice	Present	By contract	For some individuals, but not major purpose
Nursing services for community or targeted population	Emphasis upon underserved populations	Emphasis upon underserved populations	Not necessarily underserved populations
Student learning opportunities	Present	By contract	Not stated
Research and testing of theories	Present	By contract	Not stated
Generation of income	For school	For agency operation	For individual and enterprise operation

athletes; and (3) prenatal classes, relaxation sessions, and parenting programs. Clients who benefit from the center's services may be referred by a physician, social services, the school, or they may be self-referred (Riesch, 1983; Riesch, et al., 1980).The academic nursing center associated with the Catholic University of America School of Nursing serves the community by providing home visitation services, community health education, a health maintenance and socialization program for senior citizens, referral services, and a walk-in clinic. Activities of the walk-in clinic include blood pressure screening, nutrition counseling, medication teaching, stress management programs, first aid, and referral services (Ossler et al., 1982).

The Lehman College Nursing Program Nursing Center in the Bronx, New York serves the Lehman College community. The center provides health assessment and screening activities, health-related workshops, physical exams, and information and referral services (Mezey & Chiamulera, 1980).

The Clemson University Nursing Center offers primary care and wellness services to the community. Health screening and assessments, individual and family counseling, and health information and support activities are provided by the students and faculty of the Nursing College (Bagwell, 1987; Barger, 1986).

The Yale Nurse-Midwifery Practice is an academic nursing center affiliated with Yale University School of Nursing. The center provides comprehensive gynecologic and obstetrical nursing care that includes full maternity care, well-woman gynecologic care, and family planning services (Nichols, 1985).

The Erie Family Health Center, Inc., in Chicago, is an independently operated nursing center that provides primary care to individuals of all ages. Services include health assessment and education activities, wellness care, and follow-up care (Lang,1983).

The Pine Street Inn is a community-based nursing center located in Boston. The center provides health care and shelter services for the homeless that include health assessments and screening, treatment for actual health problems (head lice, trauma, exposure to heat and cold), referrals, and counseling. The comprehensive health care services provide the homeless with access to the health care system, and for many clients, Pine Street Inn is their only source of health care (Lenehan et al., 1985).

The Madison Geriatric Clinic in Madison, Wisconsin is a hospital-based nursing center that serves older adults in an outpatient setting. The comprehensive health care services include assessments, care for chronic conditions, health education, counseling, and coordination of home health and long-term institutional care (Lamper-Linden, Goetz-Kulas, & Lake, 1983).

The Nursing Home Care Unit at the Veterans Administration Medical Center in Tuskegee, Alabama, is a hospital-based center that provides rehabilitation services for chronically ill and disabled individuals. Clients who benefit from the center's services are at the post-acute/pre-independent living phase on the health–illness continuum (Nelson, 1984).

The literature reveals that a variety of nursing services are provided by all types of nursing centers (e.g., academic-based, community-based, hospital-based, and freestanding centers). The services reflect a nursing perspective, and they are aimed toward meeting the health care needs of an otherwise underserved population.

NURSING SERVICES OF PRIVATE PRACTICE

In the study of private practice nursing, eight different types of practices were identified for responses, and of these, nurse participants indicated that one or more types of service were provided. The majority of nurses indicated that they were offering consultation (53.4%), followed by counseling (46.6%), and direct client/home services (41.4%) (Table 2).

The services that were offered by the least number are legal (4.9%) and clinic (13.4%). Legal services are highly specialized and the selection of the term *clinical service* may have been misleading.

The comparison of services offered by nursing centers to private practice nursing is almost impossible. One gains the impression, however, that the services provided in private practices may be more diverse, and in some cases, directed more toward institutions and the providers of nursing services.

ORGANIZATIONAL STRUCTURE OF NURSING CENTERS

The organizational structure of a nursing center is the framework that determines the line of communication and networking among individuals and positions, the distribution of power, the allocation of resources, and the locus of decision making as related to the center's function. Several factors influence the type of organizational structure that best meets the needs of a particular center. These factors include the center's purpose, the needs of the clientele, the services rendered, and the characteristics of the staff (American Nurses' Association, 1987).

Elements commonly part of the organizational structure include a board of directors or advisory board, a director who functions as the chief executive officer, the staff who provide the center's services, and consultants. In addition, centers that are affiliated with a parent institution, (i.e., health department, hospital, or university), have an organizational structure that is consistent with the goals, philosophy, and governance of that institution.

Table 2
Types of Services Offered to Clients by Nurses in Private Practice

Type of Service	Number of Responses	Percent
Consultation	195	53.4
Counseling	170	46.6
Direct client/home services	151	41.4
Client education	142	38.9
Nursing continuing education	129	35.3
Other	95	26.0
Clinic	49	13.4
Legal	18	4.9

The board of directors or advisory board is usually comprised of professional nurses, consumers, community leaders, and other allied health professionals (Hawkins et al., 1984; Herman & Krall, 1984; Jones, 1976; Riesch, 1980). It is desirable that the board is cognizant of the contributions of nursing to health care and is knowledgeable about and supportive of nursing service (American Nurses' Association, 1987). The advisory board that serves the Nursing Center at the University of Wisconsin, Milwaukee, functions like many boards in that it advises nursing center staff, links community needs with nursing center resources, and evaluates the center's programs and activities (Riesch, Felder, & Stauder, 1980).

The chief executive officer or director of the nursing center is responsible for providing direction for the center's operation and its integration into the community. In addition, the directory manages the administration of the center, acquires and allocates resources, provides leadership for personnel, participates with the board to determine and achieve the center's goals, and oversees, evaluates, and revises the center's goals and activities (American Nurses' Association, 1987).

The staff of the nursing center include those individuals who directly provide the center's services or assist in the delivery of services. The center's goals, purpose, resources, and clientele influence the selection of staff. Staff may be employed by the director of the nursing center, the parent institution, (i.e., hospital or university), or they may be contracted for their services. Providers of care for academic-based nursing centers are usually faculty and students (Barger, 1986b). Contracted service providers include nutritionists, dietitians, social workers, physicians, nurse practitioners, and speech and physical therapists (Bagwell, 1987; Herman & Krall, 1984). Other staff who serve to compliment the nursing center include administrative, maintenance and computer personnel, clerical workers, and various technicians (American Nurses' Association, 1987).

Nursing center consultants provide valuable support and guidance. Professional nurses, lawyers, and physicians often provide consulting and collaborative services that enhance the center's ability to achieve its goals. For example, the Nursing Center, located at the University of Wisconsin, Milwaukee, consults with a local physician who acts as liaison between the center and the medical community (Barger, 1986b).

In summary, the organizational structure of the nursing center is the framework that determines the locus of decision making, the networking among individuals, the distribution of power, and the allocation of resources. Although no organizational structure is ideal for all nursing centers, it is desirable that the organizational structure works to enhance collegiality and collaboration among nurses and other professionals (American Nurses'

Association, 1987). Furthermore, it is important that the organizational structure is effective in achieving the goals of the nursing center.

ORGANIZATION OF PRIVATE PRACTICE

Three organizational models for private practice for nursing service were apparent from the study: the solo practice model, the group practice model, and the nursing service organization model

The solo practice model involves the practice of one professional nurse who formally establishes a practice to provide nursing services for a selected group of clientele. The nursing service may be general or specialized and may include direct services and case management, or both.

The group practice model is the provision of nursing services by two or more professional nurses who formally organize to render nursing services to a population. They share equipment, space, and personnel, and distribute the income in keeping with prior agreements regarding their investment and distribution of earnings. The group practice may represent a single nursing specialty, or multiple nursing specialties, or a generalized type of nursing practice. Again, the service may be a direct service or case management, or both.

The nursing service organization model is structured to provide nursing services to a population or related services to professionals and health care institutions, or both. The nursing service organization model may involve investments by individuals other than professional nurses, and earned income is distributed in accordance with agreements made at the time of investment. The services provided may be direct client services of a generalized or specialized type, or they may be a service to enable an institution to perform nursing services or enhance nursing services.

The three models vary in locus of control, level of staff, locus of decision making, and degree of professional autonomy exercised by the practitioner (Table 3).

OWNERSHIP, FINANCIAL STATUS, LEGAL STRUCTURE, AND AUTONOMY

Academic nursing centers, community nursing centers, and private practice enterprises can be compared on a set of variables that relate to ownership, financial status, legal structure, and degree of autonomy. The three types of

Table 3
Comparison of Organizational Models

Type of Model	Locus of Control	Level of Staff	Locus of Decision Making	Degree of Prof. Autonomy
Solo Practice	Professional nurse (owner)	Professional nurse	Professional nurse (owner)	High
Group Practice	Professional nurses (partners)	Professional nurses	Professional nurses (partners)	High
Nursing Service Organization	Board of directors, stockholders	Mixed	Board of directors, stockholders	Variable

nursing centers differ in ownership and financial status (Table 4). The legal form of the academic and community centers is either a professional or a business corporation. In private practice, an owner may choose a sole proprietorship, a partnership, or a professional or business corporation. Autonomy in all three types may be high or varied, depending on the role of the board and stockholders, if these are part of the form.

FUTURE MODELS FOR NURSING CARE DELIVERY[3]

One of the major changes that has taken place in the health care delivery system has been concerned with the financing of health care. The economic environment has led to a reexamination of the financing and structuring of organizations, and the means of relating these so that care is affordable. The principles of providing capitation as the basis for payment, and the use of prospective payment predominate the current thinking of policymakers. For nurses engaged in practice, these two principles should be considered in any discussions relating to reimbursement for nursing services. Nurses in practice should develop systems and the necessary structures that will provide nursing services for an enrolled population for a fixed payment, calculated on a fixed schedule of fees or on a per-capitation basis. Adaptations of the health maintenance organization (HMO) models, preferred provider organization (PPO) models, and independent physicians association (IPA) models are in

---

[3]The following sections are taken from Aydelotte, Hardy, & Hope (1988).

Table 4
Comparison of Nursing Centers and Private Practice
Enterprises on Three Variables

Variables	Academic Nursing Center	Community Nursing Center	Private Practice Enterprise
Organizational Ownership	College or school within educational institution	Community agency or sub-unit in agency	Individual nurse or group of individuals as partners or stockholders
Financial Status	Non-profit	Non-profit	Usually for profit
Legal Form or Structure	Corporation, incorporated	Corporation, incorporated	Sole proprietor-ship or partner-ship or corpora-tion
Autonomy	High	Varied, depends on role of board of directors and its composition	Sole proprietor-ship and pro-fessional cor-poration, high business cor-poration, varies

order. The populations that are to be considered for enrollment are numerous. For example, there are nurses who are caring for the homeless, the aged, the mentally ill, young families, and women. Through a marketing analysis, the population and services needed can be defined. An analysis will also illuminate the opportunity that is present.

The Independent Professional Nurses Association

An adaptation of the IPA model may be the simplest form since it does not interrupt the individual nurse's practice style. Nurses in private practice in a community voluntarily join together in an association and contract with other organizations to provide nursing services to a defined population. For example, nurses who are in solo practice or in a small-group practice would organize an IPNA (Independent Professional Nurses Association). Other organizations, for example, businesses, schools, hospitals, or other provider groups or individual subscribers, would pay the IPNA a prospective payment for a set benefit package for their employees. For example, the benefit package could include units of service of home health services, health promotion, health maintenance, stress management, or specialized services, such as rehabilitation or intensive nursing services. The benefit package would be negotiated in relation to the competence and skills of the nurses in the IPNA, the needs of the population to be served, and the organization payers or the subscribers. The prospective payment is made by the organization to the IPNA, who reimburses the nurses on a schedule that is negotiated in advance (Figure 1).

The reimbursement of the nurse rendering the nursing service is less than the agreed schedule payment, since cost of operating the IPNA, which serves as the financial intermediary, and the accumulation of a reserve are usually necessary.

The advantages of an IPNA may not at first be readily seen, but there are a number. First, because the IPNA represents a collective that can provide a more comprehensive nursing service, the IPNA may promote negotiation of contracts with organizations. Second, the panel of nurses comprising the IPNA offers a choice of nurse provider to the enrollees needing the nursing service, and moreover, that choice may well be a nurse from whom the enrollee has received prior service. Third, the existence of a panel of nurses assures continuity of nursing services if a solo nurse provider is unable to meet the need of an enrollee or if a referral to another type of nurse provider is in order. Finally, such a plan does not erode the private relationship that may have already been developed.

Preferred Professional Nurse Provider

The second model that should be considered is the adaptation of the PPO. Reference to this type of organization has already appeared in the nursing literature. Collins defined PPO as "a combination of fee-for-service and prospective payment. The health-care provider contracts with the consumer

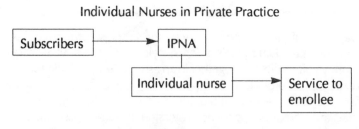

Figure 1
Nurses in IPNA: Payment and Service Flow

for an agreed upon, discounted price" (Collins, 1987, p. 86). A preferred nurse provider organization (PNPO) would consist of a professional nurse practice group contracting with an employer, such as a business owner, a nursing home operator, a school board, insurers, or a hospital board, to provide comprehensive nursing services for a fixed schedule of fees for a fixed population. The contract is direct, with no fiscal intermediary as in the INPA or in an HMO (Figure 2).

The PNPO would have these features:

- A professional nurse or a panel of professional nurses in group practice
- A set of nursing services to be provided
- A prenegotiated fee for a fixed period of time
- A legal contract to provide nursing services for the group to be served
- A mechanism for reviewing the utilization of services and quality rendered
- Use of the primary nurse concept or the nurse manager of care

The individual for whom the contract provides nursing services has no obligation to use the PNPO. In this sense, it continues the concept of freedom of choice.

In the survey of private practice, 142 individuals indicated that they were receiving referrals through contracts. One can then assume that the PNPO is already emerging as a model of practice in nursing.

Nursing Service Organization

The adaptation of the HMO is more complex than the modification of the IPA or PPO, but the resulting model has the attractive features of control by professional nurses and the direct business relationship with the enrollees. This model includes a defined population of voluntarily enrolled members

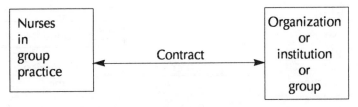

Figure 2
Preferred Nurse Provider Organization

who make payment for nursing services in advance of the need for the services. Payments are for a specific period of time, for a set benefit package. The nurses provide direct services to the enrollees and serve as case managers for them. The nurses make referrals to other health medical providers as indicated.

The structure of the NSO consists of three units: an NSO Foundation, Inc., an NSO Services, and a group nursing practice model.

The NSO Foundation, Inc., is established as a non-profit corporation for collection of enrollee payments. NSO Services is owned by the NSO Foundation for conducting marketing, collection of fees, and carrying out the business and administration services, and to contract with the nurses in group practice to provide the nursing services offered in the benefit package (Figure 3).

The NSO Foundation, a non-profit organization, is established by professional nurses who comprise its board of directors. The concept of nurses engaged in such an effort may be new to many, but, because of the changing demographics in our population, including changes in family structure and arrangements, the opportunity for providing comprehensive nursing services is real. The survey of nurses in private practice indicated that 91.8 percent of the respondents reported that clients paid for services. Furthermore, 54 percent stated that they were paid by private health insurance. It is reasonable to expect that if the opportunity were presented, children of the elderly, the healthy elderly, the young family first entering parenting, and the family where the single parent or both parents are employed, would welcome a prepaid plan, at a reasonable rate, for case management of their health needs and comprehensive nursing services. Weight Watchers, Inc., has enjoyed success as a for-profit enterprise. Professional nursing services, if carefully developed as an NSO, could enjoy the same success.

In summary, the NSO includes these features:

- A voluntarily enrolled population of members
- Prepayment by the members, set fees for services during a fixed period

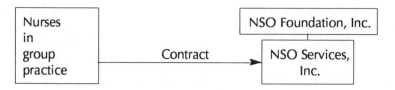

Figure 3
Nursing Service Organization

of time; the amount of the payment includes capitation and an agreed schedule for specific units of nursing services
- A basic benefit package that includes case management of care and units of direct service
- Nursing services by professional nurses with referrals to outside providers as necessary to obtain services not included in the basic benefit package

ISSUES RELATED TO NURSING CENTERS

A number of points are pertinent to the establishment of nursing centers and private practice regardless of setting. In the conduct of any enterprise, certain conditions must be present. The establishment of the enterprise is based upon the assessment of the community to learn if an opportunity for selling the service truly exists.

The decision to offer a service rests on whether or not there is a market for it. The decision requires knowledge of the community, knowledge of the potential that nursing service offers, and knowledge of resources. Wise planning and risk are involved, but above all, the ability to forecast the results of the undertaking is essential. All individuals and groups considering the establishment of an enterprise would benefit by studying the American Nurses' Association pamphlet, *Nursing Centers: Concept and Design* (1987).

In academic nursing centers, there are a number of special issues:

- Are all faculty members expected to participate in the center?
- How are faculty loads and expectations of the faculty role changed if the faculty member participates?
- How does participation in center activities count in promotion and tenure decisions?
- What are the rewards for participation? Are they financial? Are teaching loads reduced?
- How are commitments to the service aspect met on weekends, holidays, and vacations, and between academic periods? The overriding concern must be service, or clientele will dissipate.

In community centers, the issues are slightly different, although one of the issues is the means of providing continuity of services. Continuity of service is essential in building the confidence of the clientele and the community. Major problems in all centers and in private practice are the building of referral patterns, the handling of competition from other providers, and reimbursement. The problem of reimbursement will require the energies and wisdom of all of us. The interpretation of what nursing really is, what it provides, and how it must be financially rewarding, is a challenge for us.

REFERENCES

American Nurses' Association. (1987). *The nursing center: Concept and design.* Kansas City, MO: Author.

Arlton, D., & Miercort, A. (1980). A nursing clinic: The challenge for student learning opportunities. *Journal of Nursing Education, 19*(1), 53–58.

Aydelotte, M. K., Hardy, M. A., & Hope, K. L. (1988). *Nurses in private practice: Characteristics, organizational arrangements, and reimbursement policy.* Kansas City, MO: American Nurses' Association.

Bagwell, M. A. (1987). Client satisfaction with nursing center services. *Journal of Community Health Nursing, 4*(1), 29–42.

Baird, S., & Benner, R. (1985). Keeping a university well with a health promotion clinic. *Nursing and Health Care, 6*(2), 107–109.

Barger, S. (1986a). Nursing center: From concept to reality. *Journal of Community Health Nursing, 3*(4), 175–182.

Barger, S. (1986b). Academic nurse-managed centers: Issues of implementation. *Family and Community Health, 9*(1), 12–22.

Breckinridge, M. (1981). *Wide neighborhoods: A story of the frontier nursing service.* Lexington, KY: University Press of Kentucky.

Collins, B. A. (1987). Nursing PPO's for corporate clients. *Nursing Economics, 5*(3), 86–89.

Culbert-Hinthorn, P., Fiscella, K., & Shortridge, L. (1985). A nurse-managed clinical practice unit: Part I—the positives. *Nursing and Health Care, 6*(2), 97–100.

Douglas, E. T. (1970). *Margaret Sanger: Pioneer of the future.* New York: Holt, Rinehart & Winston.

Duffy, D., & Halloran, M. C. (1986). Meeting the challenges of academic roles through a nursing center practice model. *Journal of Nursing Education, 25*(2), 55–58.

Fehring, R., Schulte, J., & Riesch, S. (1986). Toward a definition of nurse-managed centers. *Journal of Community Health Nursing, 3*(2), 59–67.

Grimes, D., & Stamps, C. (1980). Meeting the health care needs of older adults through a community nursing center. *Nursing Administration Quarterly, 4*(3), 31–40.

Hall, L. E. (1963). A center for nursing. *Nursing Outlook, 11*(11), 805–806.

Hauf, B. J. (1977). An evaluative study of a nursing center for community nursing student experiences. *Journal of Nursing Education, 16*(8), 7–11.

Hawkins, J., Igou, J., Johnson, E., & Utley, Q. (1984). A nursing center for ambulatory, well, older adults. *Nursing and Health Care, 5*(4), 209–212.

Henry, O. M. (1978, October). Demonstration centers for nursing practice, education, and research. Paper presented at the annual meeting of the American Public Health Association, Los Angeles, CA.

Herman, C., & Krall, K. (1984). University sponsored home care agency as a clinical site. *Image, 16*(3), 71–75.

Hodgins, E., & Smith, M. J. (1925). Centralization of nursing in Cleveland. *American Journal of Nursing, 25*(3), 173–175.

Jones, A. (1976). Overview of a nursing center for family health services in Freeport. *Nurse Practitioner, 1*(6), 26–31.

Kinlein, M. L. (1972). Independent nurse practitioner. *Nursing Outlook, 20*(1), 22–24.

Lamper-Linden, C., Goetz-Kulas, J., & Lake, R. (1983). Developing ambulatory care clinics: Nurse practitioners as primary providers. *Journal of Nursing Administration, 13*(12), 11–18.

Lang, N. M. (1983). Will they survive? *American Journal of Nursing, 83*(9), 1291–1293.

Lenehan, G., McInnis, B., O'Donnell, D., & Hennessey, M. (1985). A nurses' clinic for the homeless. *American Journal of Nursing, 25* (3), 1237–1240.

Mezey, M., & Chiamulera, D. (1980). Implementation of a campus nursing and health information center in the baccalaureate curriculum. *Journal of Nursing Education, 19*(5), 7–10.

Nelson, D. (1984). Nurse managed rehabilitation. *Nursing Management, 15*(3), 30–39.

Nichols, C. (1985). Faculty practice: Something for everyone. *Nursing Outlook, 33*(2), 85–90.

Ossler, C., Goodwin, M., Mariani, M., & Gilliss, C. (1982). Establishment of a nursing clinic for faculty and student clinical practice. *Nursing Outlook, 30*(7), 402–405.

Riesch, S. K. (1983). The Nursing Center: UW-Milwaukee. *The Leading Edge, 3*(2), 1–4.

Riesch, S. K. (1987). Profiles of nursing centers. Unpublished paper.

Riesch, S., Felder, E., & Stauder, C. (1980). Nursing centers can promote health for individuals, families, and communities. *Nursing Administration Quarterly, 4*(3), 1–8.

Wahlquist, G. (1984). Impact of a nurse managed clinic in multiple sclerosis. *Journal of Neurosurgical Nursing, 16*(4), 193–196.

2

The Historic Origins of Nursing Centers

Laurie K. Glass,PhD, RN, FAAN

This chapter depicts the historical origins of nursing centers. By exploring the historical roots of current concepts we can refresh our memory as to what did or did not work; stimulate new ideas; facilitate our decision making; and encourage ourselves to proceed where previous successes are evident. There has been a recent resurgence in nursing centers. There are numerous academic-based and independent nursing centers, and legislation creating community nursing organizations recently was passed.

Nursing centers are a way to deliver nursing services; they will be placed within the context of the types of service delivery known since the beginning of organized nursing. Who works in the center, or out of the center as the case may be, is an important aspect of this history. The decisions about title, definition, scope of practice, and the type of work that nurses did tells us something about how we got to where we are today. Finally, four excellent examples of nursing centers that were in existence prior to 1930 will be described. No attempt has been made to be exhaustive in presenting nursing centers in this paper. I will concentrate on activities prior to 1940 and be selective about examples. The research needed for this paper represents only a beginning for the search for one piece of our history.

MODES OF NURSING SERVICE DELIVERY

The origins of modern nursing date back to 1873. This year marks the creation of the first Nightingale schools in the United States and is generally used by historians as a starting point. In the last two decades of the nineteenth century, there were few actual roles for nurses. Goodnow (1923, 1934) provided a simple framework for the delivery of nursing services during that time. She divided it into hospital nursing, private (duty) nursing, and visiting nursing. Hospital nursing and private nursing involved graduate nurses caring for affluent paying patients. Private nursing could be further described as hourly nursing or group nursing, depending on whether a nurse stayed for just a few hours, or was caring for two or more patients in a hospital setting. It was estimated that about 10 percent of the population, largely the upper classes, received nursing services in this manner (Goodnow, 1934). Visiting nursing delivered nursing services to the poor, usually under the sponsorship of some group or individual. Visiting nursing, also called "district nursing", provided care for another 10 percent of the population. It is the concept of visiting nursing that eventually led to public health nursing; and it is public health nursing that leads us to the concept of nursing centers. A look at visiting nursing at the turn of the century will provide the historical context of this belief.

However, before proceeding with an in-depth look at visiting and public health nursing, I need to clarify the rationale for the provision of services for only 20 percent of the population, noticed in the early 1930s. The 80 percent that were left unserved were defined as "the middle class" who received care in their own homes by relatives and untrained nurses. "Household nursing" was the term used to describe a new role for nurses, that is, trained nurses who supervised and taught others to care for this group in their homes (Goodnow, 1934).

Visiting nursing has its origins in the resurgence of humanitarianism that occurred at the turn of the century. All of the resulting social service-type activities that emerged at that time first appeared in London, and gradually drifted to the United States. These included the settlement house movement, and the YWCA and YMCA. In the United States, the YMCA started in 1851 to develop the spiritual, social, physical, and intellectual well-being of men. The YWCA began in 1866 with the same goals for women. Jane Addams, who had been in London, initiated the settlement house movement in the United States in 1889 with Hull House in Chicago.

The first known visiting nurse in the United States was sent out in 1877 by the Women's Branch of the New York City Mission (Kalisch & Kalisch, 1986). A couple of years later the New York Ethical Society placed nurses in city dispensaries, and in 1886 the Boston Instructive Nursing Association was organized to promote health education. By 1890, there were 21 organizations engaged in the work of visiting nursing, most of them with no more than one nurse (Kalisch & Kalisch, 1986).

Visiting nurse services originated from many different groups. The following examples give an idea of the types of groups that might have sponsored a visiting nurse: Mrs. Ranyard's Bible and Domestic Mission; the National Association for Providing Trained Nurses for the Sick Poor; the Ladies Benevolent Society; the Lying-In Charity for Attending Indigent Women in their Homes; and the Milk and Baby Hygiene Association (Dolan, 1963).

A well-known model that developed for visiting nursing was "the settlement", popularly depicted by the Nurses Settlement on Henry Street in New York City. As Goodnow stated in 1923, "settlement work was coming into general notice, it followed naturally that nurses themselves should organize similar enterprises" (p. 193). While Lillian Wald was the first to organize in 1893, there were other nurse-managed settlement houses, for example: Miss Cabaniss and Miss Minor in Richmond, Virginia, in 1901; Miss Octavine Briggs in San Francisco, in 1900; Miss Elizabeth Ashe also in San Francisco, in 1903; Miss Margaret H. Pierson in Orange, New Jersey, in 1900; and Miss Lydia Holman in the North Carolina Mountains (Goodnow, 1923, p. 193–194; "The Development," 1906, pp.35–51).

Before proceeding with the transition to public health nursing, a definition is offered by the Committee for the Study of Nursing Education in the Goldmark Report (1923): "visiting or district nursing is the care of the sick in their homes by trained nurses" (p. 41). To be more descriptive, also consider Lee's (1893) statement, ". . . where there are no proper appliances, and where the nurse can rarely see the doctor—in some cases not at all" (p. 130). The difference between private-duty nursing and visiting nursing was that the nurse made daily visits rather than stay at the house, and the visits included patient and family instruction in caring for the patient during the nurse's absence.

The transition to the term "public health nursing" occurred in the early 1900s. In 1912, when the National Organization for Public Health Nursing was created, the title "public health nurse" was chosen rather than "visiting nurse" because it was more inclusive (Kalisch & Kalisch, 1986, p. 287). Lavinia Dock claimed that Lillian Wald was the first person to use the term "public health nursing" adding "public" to Florence Nightingale's term "health nursing" (Lillian Wald, 1971, p. 660). Nightingale (1893) defined health as "not only to be well, but to be able to use well every power we have" (p. 26). She defined nursing as "putting us in the best possible conditions for nature to restore or to preserve health—to prevent or to cure disease or injury" (p. 26). Evidently, Wald wished to broaden this definition, as her vision of nursing services was that services be as widely available and as effective as possible with state and federal health services. For Wald, the difference in visiting nurse associations and public health nursing agencies was that the interests in nursing work and civic work were unified in public health nursing.

Nightingale would have agreed with Wald. For Nightingale had this to say:

> The health of the unity is the health of the community. Unless you have the health of the unity there is no community health. Competition, or each man for himself . . . is the enemy of health. Combination [used like cooperation] is the antidote-combined interests, recreation, combination to secure the best air, the best food, and all that makes life useful, healthy and happy. There is no such thing as independence. As far as we are successful, our success lies in combination (p.35–36).

It sounds as if Nightingale is describing a basic concept of public health: cooperation for happy living in a healthy environment.

There was a rapid growth of organizations providing public health nursing between 1901 and 1921. In 1901 there were 58 organizations employing 130 nurses; in 1914 there were 1,992 known organizations employing 5,152 nurses; and by 1921 there were 4,024 organizations employing 11,000 nurses (Committee, 1923). Even this wasn't enough. "In order to meet generally accepted standards we should have approximately 50,000 public health nurses to serve the population of the United States" (Committee, 1923, p. 8).

This increase in the number of agencies coincides with a trend to add nurses to state health department staffs. Until 1907, no state recognized public health nurses as legitimate employees of official health or education agencies. While there were experimental programs in Los Angeles in 1898, and in New York City in 1902, Alabama was the first state to pass a County Health Law in 1907 that defined nurses as necessary employees to accomplish the work of a county health department (Kalisch & Kalisch, 1986). By 1924, half of the approximately 4,000 agencies (employing half of all public health nurses) were official branches of federal, state, county, or municipal government (Kalisch & Kalisch, 1986). This government interest was to have an effect on the practice of the public health nurse.

THE NURSE

As the title of nurse changed so did the descriptions of who she was and what she did. According to Lees, in 1893 the district nurse was to nurse the sick back to health, to cheer and brighten the home, to teach the "patient's friends how to keep the room in nursing order", and "to teach the poor those sanitary laws which are household words with the well-to-do and how they can beautify or improve their surroundings with the things they possess" (p. 131). In order to do this "a district nurse must have a real love for the poor and a real desire to lessen the misery she may see among them, and such tact as well as skill that she will do what is best for her patients, even against their will"

(Lees, 1893, p. 131). A few years later as the change to the title of public health nurse occurs, a change in the function and definition also occurs. The National Public Health Association had a rather concise definition of public health nursing: "extended and glorified visiting nursing with teaching as its important feature" (Goodnow, 1934, p. 453).

The committee that issued the Goldmark report was originally convened to study the state of public health nursing. They eventually studied the entire profession and its educational system and issued their report, *Nursing and Nursing Education in the United States* in 1923. This report contains a wealth of information about public health nursing. They defined the public health nurse as "any graduate nurse who serves the health of the community, with an eye to the social as well as medical aspects of her function, by giving bedside care, by teaching and demonstration, by guarding against the spread of infections, insanitary practices, etc" (Committee, 1923, p. 43).

At the turn of the century, in addition to discussion about what the nurse should be called, there was also a great deal of discussion and debate about what she should do. What was her scope of practice? From all evidence, the work involved the patient, the family ("its culture and characteristics"), the environment which could be tenement or rural, resources such as milk stations, city officials such as truant or police officers, and labor union officials because of sweat shop or child worker problems. Wald summarized the nurse as responsible "not only for the care of the sick, but to seek out the deep-lying basic causes of illness and misery, to protect and to prevent, that there may be in the future less sickness to nurse and to cure" (p. 21). In addition, the nurse was to educate the people, translating into simple terms the message of the expert and the scientist; realizing "she is not only serving the individual, but promoting the interests of collective society" (Wald, 1913, p. 22–23).

Wherever the nurse was practicing it is clear that the scope of her practice was broad. Whether she was working in a school, courtroom, industry, settlement, nursery, or dispensary, she was involved in "social work of a neighborly character combined with nursing" ("The Development," 1906, p. 47). The skills needed to carry on were diverse, and probably would be considered outside the realm of nursing today. The nurses did whatever was needed to fulfill their mission which was viewed within the perspective of societal need and civic development. This led to some interesting requests for the training programs. In all seriousness, Ashe recommended in 1906 that "hospital training for a district nurse include knowledge of farming, camp cooking, and dancing, as well as care of the sick" ("The Development," 1906, p. 46).

The breadth of the scope of practice did lend itself to debate with physicians. Most of this debate occurred before states had registration laws, so lists of who did what were not available. Some physicians thought the public health nurse should carry out medical procedures including resuturing wounds, while other physicians complained "there was nothing left for the doctor to do" (Foley, 1913, p. 451). To rectify the situation somewhat, the Chicago Visiting Nurses Association in 1912 compiled a list of standing orders to be used by staff nurses, for example, in the case of a patient with typhoid fever: cleansing bath, low S.S. enema P.R.N., sponge for R.T. 102.5, milk diet, emphasize need of plenty of fresh air and cold drinking water (boiled if possible), and disinfection of stools (Foley, 1913).

There were orders for 11 medical problems and 4 surgical problems. Eventually the VNA hoped to have the orders approved by the Chicago Medical Association so there would be no question as to what the nurses were doing. It is interesting to note the nurses' rationale for including "baths" in the standing orders: ". . . many patients who object strenuously to being clean in cold weather, will accept a bath philosophically when told that 'the doctor ordered it'" (Foley, 1913, p. 452).

In the early 1920s we see the first discussions about whether public health nurses should perform bedside care. Two distinct types of public health nursing are described in the Goldmark Report (Committee, 1923): "that in which the nurse confines herself to the teaching of hygiene, and that in which such instructive work is combined with the actual care of the sick" (p. 8). It is noted that this debate occurred about the same time that governmental agencies employed half of all public health nurses in the country. A relationship is obvious when considering the Goldmark Report's statement:

> The arguments for purely instructive service rests mainly on two grounds, the administrative difficulties involved in the conduct of private sick nursing by official health agencies, and the danger that the urgent demands of sick nursing may lead to the neglect of preventive educational measures which are of more basic and fundamental significance (Committee, 1923, p. 9).

The Committee (1923), chaired by C. E. A. Winslow, believed that "the combined service of teaching and nursing would yield the largest results" (p. 9). We know from our experiences today that there eventually was a split in the functions: bedside care was carried out by "visiting nurses" and educational measures were the responsibility of "public health nurses". The governmental agencies that were the voices originally calling for a split, employ the public health nurses, and private agencies provide nurses for the so-called "sick nursing". While this change marked the end of an era in nursing, it is best to remember the words of Ella Phillips Crandall, who in 1922, said:

> Let me remind you that . . . throughout the history of public health nursing (though it has run the gamut of health visitor, health teacher, social worker and even health *inspector*), it has its foundation first, last and always in nursing (pp. 644–645).

THE ORIGINS OF NURSING CENTERS

It is from these beginnings that nursing centers arose. The basic concept is public health nursing as defined at the turn of the century when the duties included hands-on care, teaching, and the manipulation of resources. Service access at that time was as varied as it is today—from picking up messages at a local pharmacy, being fetched by a child, giving advice at a milk station, or operating a "nurses settlement". In order to find the grandparents of today's nursing centers, I sought some indication of a philosophy similar to the American Nurses' Association 1987 definition, that is, "organizations that give the client direct access to professional nursing services" (p. 1). I found the similarity that I sought in the words of Lillian D. Wald who said, "nurses should be at the 'call of people who needed them' without the intervention of a medical man" (Woolf, 1937). Wald is best known for her innovative and original ideas about public health nursing and her establishment of the first nurse settlement. Wald established what we today would call independent nursing practice. Wald and Mary Brewster did this, according to their colleague Lavinia Dock:

> . . . free from every form of control, "without benefit of" managers, committees, medical encouragement or police approval . . . [they went there, to Henry Street,] to do what they could do, to see what they could see and to publicize all that was wrong and remediable by making their findings known as widely as possible. ("Lillian D. Wald," 1971, p. 660).

Translated this means that Wald and Brewster did what they thought was right without asking permission and one of their ways of bringing about change was that of embarrassment. By publicizing the conditions of the neighborhood and their patients, the wealthy citizens who owned the tenements and factories were compelled to exercise their philanthropic duty. A closer look at examples of early nursing centers, will make the relationship to current practice clear.

Examples

Four examples of early models for nursing centers are described here. Two of these are nurse settlements, one located on Henry Street in New York City and the other located in Orange, New Jersey. The third example is a clinic with a specific focus in Brooklyn started by Margaret Sanger, and the final example is the country nursing service operating in the Kentucky mountains, which was the dream of Mary Breckinridge.

Most nurses have heard something about Lillian Wald (1867–1940) and her house on Henry Street. In 1893, at the age of 26, Wald established the Nurses Settlement with "no defined program other than the desire to find the sick and to nurse them, and to establish [themselves] socially in the neighborhood . . . in which they desired to work" (Wald, in "The Development," 1906, p. 36). The settlement, with nine resident nurses, moved into the house on Henry Street in 1895. The services grew quickly with an emphasis on nursing, social, and educational activities. In 1905 the nurses cared for 5,032 patients in their homes, making 43,503 nursing visits and 4,732 "friendly visits". In addition, there were 13,791 "first-aid treatments" given in the first aid room at the settlement house. The desire for direct access to the nurse was maintained; of the 5,032 patients, 2,398 were referred by their families, 753 were referred by charitable agencies, and 1,881 were referred by physicians ("The Development," 1906). By 1909, 37 nurses worked with supervisors at Henry Street and 10 staff nurses actually lived in the house (Kalisch & Kalisch, 1986).

The nursing services extended beyond basic visiting and first aid. The settlement nurses ran a convalescent home on the Hudson River and worked out of five other social settlements and two neighborhood tenements. In 1903, Wald was instrumental in placing nurses in the schools where in one year the number of students sent home because of a health problem dropped from 10,567 to 1,101 (Kalisch & Kalisch, 1986). In 1909 she persuaded the Metropolitan Life Insurance Company to provide nursing service for their policy holders. By the end of that year there were 14 Metropolitan Nursing Centers; by 1912 there were 589 across the country (Kalisch & Kalisch, 1986). A woman who was never short of ideas, Wald also suggested (1911) that the Red Cross, during times when there were no disasters, provide rural nursing service. This idea would eventually become the Red Cross Town and Country Nursing Service (1913).

Lillian Wald was a woman who had a clear idea of what a nurse could do and how she was to be accessed. She believed in the concept of neighborhood nursing, with nurses living in the neighborhood, getting to know the culture and characteristics of the people, and responding with appropriate services.

While the Nurse Settlement on Henry Street is probably the most well known among today's nurses, there were other nurse settlements. The Orange Visiting Nurses' Settlement in Orange, New Jersey had a particularly interesting program of services. The settlement was organized in 1900 to provide a home for the visiting nursing service that was part of the curriculum at the Orange Training School for Nurses. With the financial backing of a "friend" and a new wing on a tenement house donated by a physician, the settlement was ready for business. The house family of 12 consisted of a head worker, two graduate nurses and two pupil nurses, a graduate nurse who directed the work of the anti-tuberculosis committee, an instructor of domestic science from Simmons College, six graduate nurses engaged in private or hourly nursing, two trained attendants, a maid, and a laundress. In addition, one room was rented to a doctor who practiced in the neighborhood (Pierson, in "The Development," 1906). In 21 months (1904—1906) 9,277 visits were made by the visiting nurses. But visiting nurse service was only a small piece of the work that occurred at the settlement. The nurses also ran a day nursery, a supply closet, a first aid room, and an agency for private duty nurses; hosted lectures, receptions, and the Training School Alumni Association; and provided an orthopedic clinic, a rest room for "tired nurses", and school nurses. Pierson, the head nurse at the settlement, offered a somewhat understated summary on the house activity:

> The nurses' settlement offers a many-sided opportunity of wonderful economic value for the sharing of the fruits of professional training with suffering humanity ("The Development," 1906, p. 51)

The third example is a single focus center. Margaret Sanger 1870–1966) began her nursing career as a visiting nurse in New York City. Her actual civic involvement began with a labor strike in 1912, when she was put in charge of evacuating the children of Lawrence, Massachusetts. Sanger's involvement with poor women and children stimulated her interest in birth control and initiated her crusade for women's control over their bodies. Sanger couldn't access birth control information in the United States. Because the Comstock Act of 1873 declared birth control information as obscene matter and prohibited mailing any of it, a trip to France was necessary. In 1916, Sanger, her sister Ethel Byrne who was also a nurse, and a woman named Fania Mindell "opened the first birth control clinic in America, the first anywhere in the world except the Netherlands" (Sanger, 1971, p. 216). The clinic was located in a Brooklyn neighborhood where the flyer was printed in three languages: English, Italian, and Yiddish. They saw at least 150 women the first day (Sanger, 1971). It was a few days before an undercover policewoman appeared as a woman in need and Sanger and the others were arrested and jailed. Sanger spent 30 days in the work house; it would be the first but not the last of her arrest record.

Sanger, like Wald, had visions of what nurses should be doing for people. Jail did not deter her from her efforts to deliver the services women wanted. Sanger eventually established the American Birth Control League (1921) and the National Committee on Federal Legislation for Birth Control (1928) which was the forerunner of today's Planned Parenthood Federation. Her continued efforts to provide birth control information resulted in numerous problems for her. She was a liberated woman ahead of her time. Evidence for this statement is found in the fact that her husband cared for their children while she worked. He also was arrested while she was in exile in Europe in 1914 for doing what she told him to do. He was distributing illegal pamphlets (*Family Limitations*) on birth control (Reed, 1980). When they finally parted ways in 1920, Mr. Sanger received custody of the children.

The fourth example is the Frontier Nursing Service. In 1923, Mary Breckinridge (1881–1965) set out to determine where nursing service was needed. She surveyed a three-county area in rural, mountainous Kentucky, covering an area of 1,000 square miles and 30,000 people. She located 9 medical doctors, not all of them licensed, and 148 midwives of whom she interviewed 53 whose average age was 60.3 years (Breckinridge, 1942). Breckinridge concluded that a decentralized service was needed, the supply of licensed doctors was inadequate, the number of midwives could be reduced by three-fourths if they were young and well mounted [in horseback riding], and two attendants were necessary for each unit though not all of their time was needed for midwifery.

Based on her study, The Kentucky Committee for Mothers and Babies opened their first nursing center at Hyden, in Leslie County, in September 1925. They decided "not to look for work that month, only to take up what fell in [their] way" ("The First Centers," 1925). This didn't seem to affect their business; for the month of September, 233 patients were seen in 561 visits. This obviously was a place in need of services. The second nursing center was opened in October of that year. The name was changed to Frontier Nursing Service (FNS) in 1928. The comprehensive objectives of the service cover skilled care for sickness in all ages, and women in childbirth, the health education of the population, provision of social services, and advancement of economic independence (Frontier Nursing Service, 1938).

By 1930 there was six nursing centers (indeed called "nursing centers"), all of which were named after donors: for example, the Jesse Preston Draper Memorial Nursing Center at Beech Fork and the Frances Bolton Nursing Center at Possum Bend. Eventually there would be a small hospital at Hyden and a graduate school of midwifery (only the second in the United States).

Each nursing center served a five-mile radius, was staffed by at least two nurse midwives whose time was split at 25 percent each for maternity work, other bedside nursing, infant and preschool hygiene, and public health work including inoculations and school hygiene ("Mary Breckinridge," 1930). Until a midwifery school was started in the United States, the nurses received their midwifery training in England and Scotland. They were taught to ride and care for the horses immediately upon arrival. The Frontier Nursing Service Quarterly Bulletin included many nurse–horse stories, as it was the main mode of transportation.

It is interesting to note that for a few years there was a doctorally prepared nurse on the FNS staff: Mary R. Willaford was probably the third nurse in the United States to earn a doctorate (Brown, 1958). She received the PhD degree from Teachers College in 1932; her dissertation was titled "Income and Health in Remote Rural Areas." Willaford was listed as the Assistant Director in the 1938 *FNS Quarterly Bulletin.* There is some evidence that Breckinridge encouraged Willaford to pursue her education (Dammann, 1982).

The nursing service was supported by a prospective payment system, "subscriptions of not less than a dollar from every householder" once a year were "payable in money or in kind" ("Resolutions," 1925). The services for a delivery case or major surgery was $5 extra. Breckinridge did solicit donations of money and any supplies. In fact, a solicitation statement in the *Quarterly Bulletin* read, "Everything sent is needed and will be most gratefully received . . . " ("Directions for Shipping," 1938). The Frontier Nursing Service is an example of nurses surviving against all odds, including floods, fire, and famine. They have a long, exciting history worthy of further study.

SUMMARY

The four examples presented are representative of nursing service organizations at the turn of the century that fit our current definition of nursing center. They share commonalities that led to their creation and continuation. These nursing centers were created to respond to a recognized need: There was a clientele that was not being served; the clientele served were generally poor, of low socioeconomic status; and income generation (money) was not a motivating factor for the nurses. There was a strong leader for each center who championed the cause and took the risks, and these centers were all very successful at what they set out to do. It is interesting to note that the commonalities from the turn of the century can also be applied to the 1980s. Using this history to refresh our memory can help us build on the strong base that these early nursing centers provided.

REFERENCES

American Nurses' Association. (1987). *The nursing center: Concept and design.* Kansas City, MO: Author.

Breckinridge, M. (1942). Midwifery in the Kentucky mountains, an investigation in 1923. *The Quarterly Bulletin of the Frontier Nursing Service, 17*(4), 29–53.

Brown, A. F. (1958). *Research in nursing.* Philadelphia: W.B. Saunders.

Committee for the Study of Nursing Education. (1923). *Nursing and nursing education in the United States.* New York: Macmillan.

Crandall, E. P. (1922). An historical sketch of public health nursing. *American Journal of Nursing, 22,* 641–645.

Dammann, N. (1982). *A social history of the Frontier Nursing Service.* Sun City, AZ: Social Change Press.

The development of nurses' settlements. (1906). *Charities and the Commons, 16*(1), 35–51.

Directions for shipping. (1938). *The Quarterly Bulletin of the Frontier Nursing Service, 13*(3), 27.

Dolan, J. A. (1963). *Goodnow's history of nursing* (11th ed.). Philadelphia: W. B. Saunders.

The first centers of nurse-midwifery. (1925). *The Kentucky Committee for Mothers and Babies Quarterly Bulletin, 1*(2), 12–13.

Foley, E. L. (1913). Standing orders. *American Journal of Nursing, 13,* 451–453.

Frontier Nursing Service, Inc., its object. (1938). *The Quarterly Bulletin of the Frontier Nursing Service, 13*(3), 29.

Goodnow, M. (1923). *Outlines of nursing history* (3rd ed.). Philadelphia: W. B. Saunders.

Goodnow, M. (1934). *Outlines of nursing history* (5th ed.). Philadelphia: W. B. Saunders.

Kalisch, P. A., & Kalisch, B. J. (1986). *The advance of American nursing* (2nd ed.). Boston: Little, Brown.

Lees, F. S. (1893/1949). On district nursing. In *Nursing of the sick 1893* (pp. 127–133). New York: McGraw-Hill.

Lillian D. Wald, our first public health nurse. (1971). *Nursing Outlook, 19,* 659-660.

Mary Breckinridge, RN nurse-midwife. (1930). *American Journal of Nursing, 30,* 311–312.

Nightingale, F. (1893/1949). Sick nursing and health nursing. In *Nursing of the sick 1893* (pp. 24–43). New York: McGraw-Hill.

Reed, J. (1980). Margaret Sanger. In B. Sicherman & C. H. Green (Eds.), *Notable American women, the modern period* (pp. 623–627). Cambridge, MA: Belknap Press.

Resolutions. (1925). *The Kentucky Committee for Mothers and Babies Quarterly Bulletin, 1*(2), 15–17.

Sanger, M. (1971). *Margaret Sanger, an autobiography.* New York: Dover (reprint of 1938 ed. by W. W. Norton).

Wald, L. D. (1913). Nursing. *Survey, 31*, 355–356.

Woolf, S. J. (1937, March 7). Miss Wald at 70 sees her dreams realized. *New York Times Magazine.*

3

Survival Strategies for Community Nursing Centers

Sally Peck Lundeen, PhD, RN

The distinguishing mark of community nursing centers (CNCs) is that they offer consumers direct access to nursing services. Although many nurses believe that CNCs are a logical extension of the services that public health and community nurses have provided for decades, these centers are nonetheless being heralded by others as a new and innovative health care delivery mechanism. In either case, proponents agree to the importance of developing and carefully evaluating CNCs in order to determine what their potential is for helping consumers reach and maintain a higher level of wellness. In 1987, one group of nursing leaders operationally defined nursing centers as follows:

> Nursing centers—sometimes referred to as community nursing organizations, nurse-managed centers, nursing clinics and community nursing centers—are organizations that give the client direct access to professional nursing services. Using nursing models of health, professional nurses in these centers diagnose and treat human responses to actual and potential health problems, and promote health and optimal functioning among target populations and communities. The services provided in these centers are holistic and client-centered, and are reimbursed at a reasonable fee level. Accountability and responsibility for client care and professional practice remain with the professional nurse. Overall accountability and responsibility remain with the nurse executive.

> Nursing centers are not limited to any particular organizational configuration. Nursing centers may be freestanding businesses or may be affiliated with universities or other service institutions such as home health agencies and hospitals. The primary characteristic of the organization is responsiveness to the health needs of the population. (Aydelotte, Barger, Branstetter, Fehring, Lindgren, Lundeen, & Riesch, 1987).

Community nursing centers throughout the United States are based on various practice models, target different populations, may or may not be affiliated with academic institutions, and have a variety of organizational structures. In spite of these differences, all of these centers share the common concern of finding a solid source or sources of funding that will ensure a viable future. This chapter will review several strategies which should be considered when designing a long-term plan for the fiscal and organizational management of a community nursing center.

Many community nursing centers are faced with the complex health care problems of low-income urban or rural populations. Many of the health care needs of this target population are only partially addressed by Medicare and Medicaid entitlements. Often, families categorized as "the working poor," undocumented aliens, and others are, by definition, ineligible for third-party reimbursement programs. In addition, little support through third-party reimbursement is available for health promotion, counseling, or outreach activities, which are key intervention strategies used by many community nurses. The immediate survival of many CNCs therefore depends on the ability of nurses to develop creative and viable funding strategies.

The four strategies discussed here are based on the partial findings of a research project I conducted in 1986 (Lundeen, 1986). These strategies will focus only on the aspects of funding from nonclient revenue sources. In any successful organization, they should be combined with long-term funding sources that will allow stronger direct client-based revenue to be developed for CNCs. Since direct third-party reimbursement for services is currently denied professional nurses in many states and the low socioeconomic status of many nursing center clients precludes a reliance on fee for service mechanisms, other avenues for start-up as well as maintenance funding must be identified. When combined with other strategies, those outlined here allowed one community nursing center to survive and grow despite circumstances which might have otherwise destined the center to financial failure.

SEEK FUNDING BASED ON COMMUNITY NEED RATHER THAN AN ALTERNATIVE MODEL OF CARE DELIVERY

The development of an alternative delivery model (i.e., a community nursing center) may not hold the same inherent appeal for the general community or potential funders as it does for the innovative nurses who have conceptualized the project. It is important to have a clear plan for the project and present the goals and objectives, as well as the methods for achieving them as clearly as possible to funders; however, the emphasis given to the various aspects of the plan needs to be tailored to each specific funder. It is frequently more appropriate to request funds in terms of the need that must be addressed in the population to be served rather than focusing on the means (nursing care) to that end.

Let us assume that the overriding goal of a particular CNC project is to establish a demonstration program of care for the elderly that will provide in-home nursing visits while reducing the need for unnecessary physician visits. Although this may be an admirable goal in a cost-conscious environment, the implementation of a model which positions nurses as primary caregivers might raise serious political red flags to potential funders if the grant applicant overemphasizes this aspect of the model above all others. For example, the local United Way Board whose membership includes several prominent physicians from the community, might review a proposal framed with such an ideological/methodological slant as a project which would be difficult to fund. Presentation of the same project focusing on the unmet needs of the elderly in the community and seeking to alleviate their suffering through the delivery of community-based nursing services might receive a much more positive review from the same funding body. In the latter scenario, the control of the practice is relegated to a secondary position in the application for support.

It is important to note that the overall goal of establishing an alternative delivery mechanism which features nurse practitioners has not lost its importance to the applicants nor has it been obfuscated in the grant proposal. It has simply not been highlighted in deference to the overwhelming need demonstrated by the community for the services to be delivered. The same model would be presented quite differently to the State Nurses' Foundation in an attempt to secure funding for an evaluation of the project. The survival strategy is to understand, and then match as closely as possible, the interests, goals, and political persuasions of the potential funder.

SECURE FUNDING FROM MULTIPLE SOURCES

There are several pragmatic reasons for soliciting funds from multiple funders. Many private foundations limit annual contributions to small amounts. Grant awards in excess of $20,000 are frequently not available from local founda-tions. Awards from private foundations are usually made only on an annual basis. Some foundations are only willing to contribute on a one-time basis; others provide funding for a limit of two consecutive years. Even those willing to support agencies on an on-going basis required that a "new and innovative program" be presented each year in addition to the annual report of outcomes on the project currently funded. Therefore, in order to maintain a consistent level of funding for existing services and generate capital for expansion activities, it may be necessary to identify multiple sources of private support.

Multiple sources of funding may also allow CNCs to maintain a larger measure of control over their own destinies. Each funding source has a vested interest in those program efforts of a CNC to which they contribute. Reporting, therefore, can focus on specific program initiatives for each granting body. Although this prompts the need to prepare many different year-end summaries, it also allows the CNC to develop initiatives in a variety of specialty areas while still protecting the core of services offered to all clients. That is, funders interested in health promotion might donate to (and receive reports on) those aspects of the CNC services concerned with counseling, community education, or advocacy. These same granting agencies might be totally unconcerned about health professional education initiatives or research projects developed within the center. By presenting the center services selectively to various sources of support, it may be possible to generate a broader revenue resource base while simultaneously satisfying the criteria of several diverse funders.

Since most external funding is by definition "soft money," multiple funders can also protect the CNC against sudden and/or total financial collapse. The reliance on one source of funding can have devastating ramifications on an agency if, for some reason, that funding is suddenly terminated. The fickle nature of both private and public funds was exemplified in the 1970s when a shift in federal funding priorities forced the dramatic closure of hundreds of community mental health centers. The survival of a CNC may well rest on the ability of the organization to respond to a funding crisis by shifting reliance away from a threatened funding source to a more stable one. Such flexibility can be built into successful organizations through the acquisition of support from multiple funding sources.

The final argument for a piecemeal funding approach focuses on the increased ability of the CNC to retain governance over the development and delivery of a unique set of health care services. The potential desire by any one funding source to control center operations is tempered by the knowledge that there are other funders contributing substantially to the same program. This precludes the possibility that decisions regarding the basic philosophy of practice and utilization of resources will be made unilaterally by an external funding agency who might use the withholding of funds as leverage to alter the mission or the methods of the agency.

CENTRALIZE THE FUNDING STRATEGY AND THE PREPARATION OF GRANT APPLICATIONS

In order for the patchwork budget created by multiple funding sources to work efficiently, the details of all fiscal information must be monitored by a central administrator. While building a community nursing center with resources secured from multiple funders allows a great deal of latitude for creative program development, it also generates an abundance of administrative paperwork. Multiple funders necessitate the tracking of many different program budgets and fund accounts each year. Annual, sometimes quarterly, reports must be prepared for each funding source. Meticulous detail of accounts must be maintained due to the various fiscal year accounting periods (January–December, July–June, October–September) used by different foundations or funding agencies. The close interrelationship between the fiscal management of the CNC and revenue generation requires the nurse administrator to understand the intimate details of the operation. The assistance of a certified public accountant to establish and maintain an orderly bookkeeping system is invaluable for any CNC, but does not in any way subsume the nurse administrator's key role as fiscal manager.

Many CNCs have a board of directors or a community advisory board which may be quite active in the process of seeking necessary program resources. While such a group can play an important role in the development of a successful fundraising campaign, the strategy outlined here emphasizes the centralization of the actual grantsmanship function with the nurse administrator and perhaps a few selected colleagues. Applications for refunding must be prepared and new sources of revenue constantly identified if the CNC services are to be maintained with any measure of stability and continuity. The turn around time on many requests for proposals is very short and demands immediate attention to the details of grant proposal development. Frequently, a committee approach is simply ineffectual. In order for all new funding initiatives to be integrated successfully into an existing funding structure, the nurse administrator must maintain a key role in the decision-making process.

Finally, grant writing requires the development of a particular set of skills that improve with practice. Given the need to develop many proposals each year, it may be simply more efficient to rely on one or two individuals who have acquired the appropriate techniques. Many clinical providers show little interest in assisting in this process. They perceived their roles to be related to their area of clinical expertise and management at the programmatic level.

Since these duties demand the development of quite a different set of skills, there may be a tacit agreement that grant development fall within the role of central administration.

Although there is a strong case for the centralization of the revenue generation function, there is one limitation to this strategy if it is carried to the extreme. The preparation of many different grant applications or the negotiation of multiple contracts each year is a time-consuming and emotionally draining experience. It is appropriate for the nurse administrator to assist others in developing these skills to help prevent burnout. It is possible to work with several other staff or board members in this capacity as long as the responsibility for the overall planning and integration of the process remains centralized. This expansion of the function also serves to protect the agency over the long term. The loss of the sole successful grant seeker by a CNC can result in serious disruption to the organization.

PATIENCE AND PERSISTENCE ARE REQUIRED FOR SUCCESSFUL ACQUISITION OF RESOURCES

A final strategy in the analysis of financial resource acquisition concerns the need for persistence and patience in this complex process. The successful completion of a grant process or contract negotiations may not occur in the early days of CNC program development. If the program seeking funding is new and innovative and the organization itself is a newly developed entity, funders are likely to be cautious. In the case study referred to throughout this chapter, the first nine grant proposals submitted by the executive director to private foundations were rejected. It took patience, persistence, and a strong belief in the CNC model being developed to continue to develop proposals in the face of such a series of disappointments.

Persistence can be its own reward. After these nine rejections, funding was granted to this CNC by a prestigious local foundation. It should be noted that this funding was for a very specific aspect of the program which matched the particular mission of the foundation. It was not a grant that specifically endorsed the nurse-based model of care being developed. However, following this award, the success of the agency in acquisition of private foundation support shifted dramatically. Twenty-eight of the next 32 proposals to private foundations were funded.

Several strategies were used to build upon the initial funding success. After the first major grant from a private foundation is received, the nurse administrator should include information about the award in all subsequent grant proposals. The prestige of the agency can be enhanced in the eyes of other potential funders if recognition and support of a major foundation is acknowledged. As each new grant or contract is awarded, the name of the grantor agency should be added to information appended to future grant proposals. This is a key method of establishing the credibility and prestige of the agency in the network of potential donors. Most donors are interested in increasing the impact made by a successful agency. It is, therefore, more likely that those CNCs who already have attracted funding are likely to attract additional funding. It requires patience to persevere until initial funding is identified and persistence to continue to develop more and more proposals in order to maintain funding.

SUMMARY

The development of innovations in any area presents a myriad of challenges. The establishment of a community nursing center in a competitive health care market place is not a role for the faint of heart or those with limited motivation or energy to devote to such an endeavor. Even so, many nurses are committed to the goal of establishing CNCs as demonstration sites for experimentation with alternative structures of health care delivery in spite of the challenges and the odds. Until reimbursement mechanisms are modified to allow nurses practicing in CNCs to generate client/service-based revenue, reliance on alternative sources of funding will continue.

Several strategies have been presented here that have been identified as useful in the acquisition of financial resources for the support of a community nursing center. The strategies include: focusing on community need rather than the model of delivery when approaching potential donors; securing funds from multiple sources; centralizing the funding strategy and the preparation of grant applications; and adopting a policy of patience and persistence in seeking extramural funding. It is my hope that these strategies will assist those of you engaged in the struggle to develop community nursing centers to significantly improve the level of financial security in your center.

REFERENCES

Aydelotte, M. K., Barger, S. E., Branstetter, E., Fehring, R. J., Lindgren, K., Lundeen, S. P., McDaniel, S., & Riesch, S. K., (1987). *The nursing center: Concept and design.* Kansas City, MO: American Nurses' Association.

Lundeen, S. P. (1986). *Theory, reality, survival: Analysis of a neighborhood health center.* Unpublished doctoral dissertation. University of Illinois Health Sciences Center, Chicago.

4

Payment for Nursing Services: Issues in Policy Implementation

Marilyn Frenn,MSN, RN

BACKGROUND

The manner in which nurses have been paid in the United States has varied historically, as well as regionally, and by practice specialization (American Nurses' Association, 1977; Hartley & McKibbin, 1983; Harrington & Lempert, 1988; Physician Payment Review Commission, 1988; Poulin, 1985). Although payment mechanisms have been determined in part by federal legislation, recent trends suggest greater involvement in policies affecting nurses will occur at the state level (Aiken, 1984).

The purpose of this chapter is to describe the contexts within which payment varies, issues affecting payment for nursing services, and policy alternatives based on data collected from nurses regarding payment mechanisms in Wisconsin. A plan for policy implementation and evaluation in Wisconsin will be described.

This study was conducted as part of coursework supported in part by an Individual National Research Service Award (NR05946-02) funded by the Center for Nursing National Institutes of Health.

LEGISLATIVE CONTEXTS AND ISSUES
AFFECTING PAYMENT OF NURSES

The American Nurses' Association (ANA) began to study the inclusion of nursing services in prepaid health care in 1936 and since has adopted at least 20 resolutions related to third-party payment and recognition of the nurse as a primary care provider (American Nurses' Association, 1984). However, legislative changes enabling direct third-party payment for nursing services have been relatively recent.

Federal coverage for nurse practitioners (NPs), certified nurse midwives (CNMs), and certified registered nurse anesthetists (CRNAs) is shown in Table 1. Except for health maintenance organizations (HMOs), coverage included direct payment to the practitioners listed.

State laws also vary in terms which types of nurses receive direct payment

Table 1
Federal Payment Mechanisms for Nursing Specialists

Payer	NP	CNM	CRNA	NPT
Medicare				
Part A	No	No	Not since 1984	?
Part B	No	No	Yes—1984 In 1989	?
HMOs	Yes	Yes	Not applicable	?
State Medicaid	Some states	36 states	8 states	?
CHAMPUS (a)	Yes	Yes	?	Yes
FEHBP (b)	7 plans	20 plans	?	?

NP	=	Nurse practitioners, masters prepared
CNM	=	Certified nurse midwives
CRNA	=	Certified registered nurse anesthetists
NPT	=	Nurse psychotherapists

? Information not included in sources cited
(a) Civilian Health and Medical Program of the Uniformed Services
(b) Federal Employees Health Benefit Program—21 plans

Sources: American Association of Nurse Anesthetists *CRNA Facts;* Department of Defense, Doc #6010.8-R; Mulinax, 1987; U.S. Congress Office of Technology Assessment, 1986.

for services. States with legislation supporting payment for nursing services are shown by specialty groups in Table 2.

Although professional nursing associations have articulated direct payment of nurses as an avenue toward more autonomous nursing practice (American Nurses' Association, 1984; La Bar, 1983; National League for Nursing, 1981), consumers and those who potentially fund payment of nurses may be concerned that nurses provide care of the quality that they are accustomed to receiving within other payment mechanisms. The endorsements of nursing associations are supported by a number of studies both in the United States and in Canada in which equal or better care delivery by nurses as compared with physicians was documented (Aaronson, 1987;

Table 2
States with Legislation Supporting Payment for Specialty Nursing Groups

CNM	Mississippi
Alaska	Montana
Maryland	Oregon
Massachusetts	Nevada
Minnesota	**CRNA**
Montana	
New Jersey	Minnesota
New Mexico	Montana
New York	
Ohio	**Nurse Psychotherapists**
Pennsylvania	California
Utah	
West Virginia	**Registered Nurses**
NP	Maryland
	New York
California	North Dakota
New Hampshire	Washington
Maryland	West Virginia

NP   = Nurse practitioners, masters prepared
CNM   = Certified nurse midwives
CRNA = Certified registered nurse anesthetists
NPT   = Nurse psychotherapists

*In addition Blue Cross/Blue Shield directly reimburses CRNAs in 8 states (American Association of Nurse Anesthetists, *CRNA Facts*).

Sources: ANA (1984); LaBar (1986).

Alfano, 1982; Brooten et al., 1986; Gilbert, 1977; Jacox, 1984; Mayes et al., 1987; Roddy & Hambelton, 1977; Spitzer, 1976; U.S. Congress Office of Technology Assessment, 1986).

However, Jacox (1984) stated that payment for nursing services is largely a political, rather than a research issue. One salient political issue is the effect that providing direct payment to nurses will have on health care costs.

The U.S. Congress Office of Technology Assessment (1986) concluded that extending coverage for the services of NPs, CNMs, as well as physicians' assistants would benefit the health status of certain segments of the population not receiving appropriate care. Although the effects on third-party costs were deemed unclear, a long-term decrease in costs was thought possible with direct nurse payment (U.S. Congress Office of Technology Assessment, 1986). This seems especially likely given that nurses are currently paid one-third to one-fifth as much as physicians (Aiken, Blendon, & Rogers, 1981; American Association of Nurse Anesthetists, 1986).

However LeRoy (1982) documented that NP cost savings may be passed on only to the medical practice or HMO, and not to the consumer. If nurses provide services to fulfill the health care needs of underserved populations, cost increases in the range of 7–15 percent also may be expected (Harahan, 1987), except when nurses and other health professionals provide services directly rather than by referral (O'Malley, 1987). In order to realize either widespread cost reductions or increased services to needy groups, the usage and effects of existing nursing payment mechanisms must be better understood.

CURRENT RESEARCH ON PAYMENT FOR NURSING SERVICES

In their study of nurse entrepreneurs, Vogel and Dolyesh (1988) found that nurses have been quite successful in developing entrepreneurial businesses and consulting firms. Readers also are referred to Bullough, Bullough, Garvey, and Allen's (1985) annotated bibliography concerning third-party payment for nurses on a national basis.

Payment for nursing services in Wisconsin was extensively described in a study commissioned by the Wisconsin Nurses Association (WNA). In this study (Lakewood Group, 1985), federal mandates for payment of nursing specialty groups were described as shotgun in nature and detrimental to overall direct payment for nursing services. No legal barriers to direct payment for nursing services were identified in Wisconsin. Major barriers were identified in individual insurance company contracts that were based on the following perceptions: (1) nurses cannot legally perform independent functions; (2) there is a lack of knowledge about what services nurses can provide; (3) the physician is viewed as the most appropriate gatekeeper for all health care services; (4) there is a lack of evidence of the marketability of nursing services; and (5) the notion exists that payment for nursing services would generate "add-on" costs (Lakewood Group, 1985).

The Lakewood Group (1985) also found that approximately 40 percent of Wisconsin businesses are self-insured and thus may be responsive to proposals from nurses demonstrating cost-effective care delivery. The survey of WNA members, however, had too few respondents for conclusive data analysis as to whether nurses experienced difficulty in receiving third-party payment or had utilized other methods of payment (Lakewood Group, 1985). Thus, further study of nurses' experiences in obtaining payment for nursing services in Wisconsin still was needed.

METHOD

The purpose of this study was to further describe the experience of nurses in Wisconsin who received direct payment for clinical nursing services. Direct payment was operationally defined as payment for clinical nursing services by clients or third-party payers other than the nurses' employers. Although several of the respondents were also paid for consultation or educational services provided to other professionals, the focus of this study was payment for nursing care provided to individuals or groups.

Since no prior data on usage of direct payment mechanisms by nurses in Wisconsin had been found in the literature, interview questions were developed to discover any forms of payment utilized by nurses, and how payment or the lack of it affected their clients and practice. Ten general informants and 28 nurses representing specific practice settings—including nurse practitioners, certified nurse midwives, certified nurse anesthetists, gerontological nurse specialists, nurses in academic nurse-managed centers, nurse psychotherapists, home care nurses, and community generalist nurses—were asked to respond to the following questions during telephone interviews (three who requested personal interviews were so interviewed):

1. Which means of payment for client services have you found available?
2. Were these means of payment satisfactory for you? For clients?
3. Please describe any other means of payment for nursing services you have heard about.
4. What assets or limitations do you see in third-party (or other) payment for nursing services?
5. What effects might third-party payment have on client utilization of nursing services?

6. If third-party payment were to be pursued further by nurses, additional data bases may be necessary. Do you keep records of client utilization, for example, time spent, type of service, or other such data?

7. Are there other questions that should have been asked, or is there other information you would like to share regarding payment for nursing services?

The response rate was 100 percent, since all persons who were asked to participate agreed to do so. Interviews were generally 15–20 minutes in length. The investigator recorded responses immediately as reported. Copies of an earlier draft of this manuscript were sent to selected respondents in each specialty to check for accuracy of the report as well as maintenance of respondent confidentiality.

Respondents

Respondents included nurses who were generally knowledgeable about payment mechanisms in nursing and nurses who were officers of nursing specialty groups eligible for payment under federal law. Random respondents provided names of specific respondents who they thought might have experience with direct payment for nursing services, even though many specific respondents thus identified were currently in salaried positions. Specific respondents included 7 CNMs, 4 gerontological nursing specialists, 4 NPs, 4 nurses working in nursing centers (NCs) associated with schools of nursing, 3 nurse psychotherapists, 2 CRNAs, 2 home care administrators, and 2 masters-prepared nurse generalists.

Since this project was done as a part of coursework, formal review for protection of respondents' anonymity was obtained upon completion of the report prior to dissemination within guidelines for previously collected data. The interview format was reviewed by two course faculty members prior to data collection. The nature of the study was explained to potential respondents prior to their consent to participate. Confidentiality of response was maintained by reporting data in aggregates without names or characteristics that might be used to identify a particular respondent.

A snowball sampling technique (Bogdan & Biklen, 1982) was used. Each respondent recommended additional nurses with experience in pursuing direct payment who could address the effects of direct payment for clinical nursing services on clients and nursing practice. As a result of this method of sampling, most nurses in the sample practiced within one metropolitan area. However, respondents in other areas of Wisconsin were identified and interviewed within each specialty category except for home care, mental health, and general practice.

Limitations

The small sample size in some respondent categories limited our ability to make generalizations about the findings of this study. The data also reflect payment for specialty nursing services provided primarily by nurses in nonacute care settings who had educational preparation beyond that required for initial licensure.

RESULTS AND DISCUSSION

Nurses in Wisconsin in a variety of specialty practices have found available payment mechanisms. Payment sources for nurses covered by federal legislation are summarized in Table 3.

NURSES COVERED BY FEDERAL PAYMENT LEGISLATION

NPs, CNMs, CRNAs, and nurse psychotherapists all had received payments by clients or third-party payers. However, third-party payment was the exception rather than the rule. Those eligible had claims left unpaid. Client needs exceeding, or not covered by, third-party payments were described by all nurses reporting such payments.

Two different HMOs were described as paying for client services based on nurse–client assessment of need. However, this too was the exception rather than the rule. Some nurses described HMOs as closed systems, while others asked to provide services for HMOs chose not to do so because of the paucity of services covered and low level of payment.

Nurses in Wisconsin within these specialties for the most part had not used federal payment mechanisms. Reasons cited included the lower level of payment provided by governmental sources for services provided by nurses rather than physicians, legally mandated physician collaboration, and lack of coverage by private insurers when identical services were provided by nurses. These reasons made usage of the physician rather than nurse provider number financially advantageous when nurses were employed in clinics, and also made independent nursing practices unfeasible. Specific examples in each practice category are described as follows.

Nurse Practitioners

The four NPs included in this category were those educationally prepared as NPs whose practice was not primarily in gerontological care or in academic

Table 3
Payment Source Utilization in Wisconsin:
Nurses Paid through Federal Mechanisms

Payer	NP	CNM	CRNA	NPT
Medicare				
Part A	No	No	Before 1984	In clinics
Part B	No	No	Yes—1989	with physician collaboration
Medicaid	No	Yes	No	As above
CHAMPUS	No	NR	No	No
Private Insurers	No	No	As hospital employees	Yes
HMOs	No	No	As hospital employees	Yes
Agency Contracts	Yes	Salary paid by physicians	Possible	Yes
Private pay	Yes	Yes	Possible	Yes
Grants	NR	NR	NR	NR

NR	=	Not reported by respondents in ths study
NP	=	Nurse practitioners, masters prepared
CNM	=	Certified nurse midwives
CRNA	=	Certified registered nurse anesthetists
NPT	=	Nurse psychotherapists

nursing centers. These NPs were predominantly in salaried positions and used their physician's provider number for insurance claims.

One nurse practitioner lost her home care provider number because she was working with a physician and there was concern about possible duplicate billing for the same service. Some insurers would not pay unless a physician's name was on the form. The fact that most NPs were in practices with physicians and are legally dependent on physicians was seen as a factor restraining direct payment for NPs.

In one case, NP charges for identical services were the same as physician's charges. In two other cases, NPs charged less (half as much, in one case) as physicians.

Therefore, because of legally mandated physician collaboration, federal payment mechanisms available to NPs have not been used in Wisconsin. Potential cost savings to consumers that might have accrued from direct payment instead have gone to physician practices.

Certified Nurse Midwives

All seven CNMs interviewed described themselves as currently or previously employed in salaried positions in clinics or with physicians. Although CNMs had obtained Medicaid payment numbers, payment for CNM services were billed through physician or clinic provider numbers. The CNM respondents did not express dissatisfaction with being paid a salary.

However, CNMs described problems with current reimbursement mechanisms in terms of independent practices for nurse midwifery. These problems included the facts that (1) private insurers often would not pay for deliveries by CNMs, therefore clients went elsewhere; (2) Medicaid payment alone was insufficient to support independent midwifery practices since CNMs are paid at 80 percent of the $450 fee allowed physicians, whose customary fees exceed $1000; (3) Medicaid payment required membership in an HMO in certain counties, and HMOs were seen as closed systems that, except in one instance, would not pay for midwifery services; and (4) Medicaid paid only for 6-week postpartum visits, and not for family-planning teaching or other services usually provided by CNMs.

Thus, the experiences of CNMs parallel those of NPs in that disparities in payment to CNMs through Medicaid, compounded by limited private payment mechanisms, made independent practice unfeasible. Any cost savings resulting from lower CNM salaries relative to physicians did not accrue to consumers, but rather to physicians or clinics employing the CNMs.

Certified Registered Nurse Anesthetists

According to the two respondents, all CRNAs in major metropolitan areas were employed by hospitals. Wisconsin was described as not yet having any insurance plans that directly pay the 350-400 CRNAs practicing at this time.

Again, any cost savings from CRNA practice accrued to hospitals, rather than directly to consumers in Wisconsin. Therefore, since in 1984 50–70 percent of anesthesia services were provided by CRNAs, who were paid one-third to one-fourth as much as anesthesiologists (American Association of Nurse Anesthetists, 1986), the cost savings are most likely substantial.

As with the other nursing specialty groups in Wisconsin who have federally authorized payment for services, but who by law must collaborate with physicians, CRNAs largely have not used these payment sources.

Nurse Psychotherapists

For the three nurse psychotherapists interviewed, direct payment by clients was the most frequent method of payment. They did not report the use of federally mandated CHAMPUS payments. Payment by some private insurers was reported by a doctorally prepared nurse, but was only available to masters-prepared nurses with physician coverage.

HMOs were reported as largely problematic for nurses due to low coverage for services, low payments to nurses, and infringements on the nature of nursing practice. Mandated physician coverage that leads nurses to work in clinics absorbed 40–60 percent of the fees generated by nurses.

One doctorally prepared nurse described payment as satisfactory, while a masters-prepared nurse said the income from independent practice was insufficient to live on. Lack of continued visitation privileges to see hospitalized patients was problematic in terms of continuity of care.

Thus, greater usage of third-party payment was reported for nurse psychotherapists than for other groups. However, direct client payments were the greater source of revenue. Income was sufficient in one of the three cases, where the nurse received payment without mandated physician coverage.

NURSES NOT COVERED BY FEDERAL PAYMENT MECHANISMS

Payment source utilization for nurses in academic nursing centers, gerontological specialists, home care, and nurse generalists is summarized in Table 4. These nurses, not covered by federal payment mechanisms, reported contracts with housing agencies, county health programs, and institutions providing employee benefits as alternate payment mechanisms. Other nurses were paid on a fee-for-service basis, sliding payment scale, or provided free nursing care. Services included primary care for individuals as well as group classes and health screenings. Specific examples in each practice setting are as follows.

Academic Nursing Centers

Payment in academic nursing centers affiliated with schools of nursing was varied. Methods included fee for service, contracted care, HMO payment, membership fees, donations, grants, and nursing services provide free of charge by students and faculty either as part of their contract with the school or as community service.

Table 4
Payment Source Utilization in Wisconsin:
Nurses Not Paid through Federal Mechanisms

Payer	Nursing Center	Gerontological Specialist	Home Care	MSN Generalist
Medicare				
Part A	No	No	NA	No
Part B	No	No	With physician order	No
Medicaid	No	No	As above	No
CHAMPUS	No	No	No	No
Private Insurers	No	No	With physician order	Yes
HMOs	1/4	No	1/2	Yes
Agency Contracts	Yes	Yes	NA	Yes
Private Pay	Yes	Yes	Yes	Yes
Grants	Yes	Yes	NR	NR

NR = Not reported by respondents in this study
NA = Not applicable

Two NCs utilized fee for service as a primary method of payment. Three NCs also contracted with other agencies to provide specific programs or services such as physical examinations, childbirth education, and cardiopulmonary resuscitation training. One NC had received payment from an HMO within the $30 per-client per-year that HMO allocated for health promotion. Two NCs were building files of claims rejected by HMOs or insurance companies.

One NC operated with membership fees. Another requested that clients make free-will donations (amount unspecified). One NC had originally purchased equipment with foundation grant moneys. Some nursing services were provided free of charge by faculty and students. In another NC, faculty practice was included as part of their contract with the school. In the remaining three NCs faculty volunteered as a community service or were paid for the particular class or service they offered.

Third-party payment was being pursued further in two NCs. Respondents advocated personal contact, involving consumers in requesting that services be covered, statewide nursing organization efforts to facilitate direct payment, and building a file of unpaid claims with which to make a case for payment with those companies who refused.

Records are kept at all NCs concerning frequency and type of client visits. Two NCs utilize forms with information requested by insurers. One NC has set up a mechanism for cross-tabulating time spent, nature of the visit, and the fee schedule. Research also has been conducted in two NCs related to nursing diagnoses utilized in those nursing practices, should nursing diagnoses be developed as a payment mechanism.

Gerontological Nurse Specialists

The four nurses interviewed who were caring for the elderly had a variety of educational backgrounds and a variety of payment mechanisms. Educational preparation included diploma, nurse practitioner, masters degree in nursing, and an earned doctorate. Payment was achieved by contracts with managers of housing for the elderly and senior centers, through grants from United Way, the Office of Aging, church-related institutions, a hospital, through private payment in a joint practice with a physician, and by salary.

The nurse who had been in joint practice with physicians expressed equivocal satisfaction with the arrangement. She stated it was difficult because there were no other nurses and it took a while to "prove a track record." In the joint practice model, nursing services were billed at $7 per 15 minutes.

The same nurse is now salaried in an adult day-care program paid for through a combination of public and private funds. She said some clients probably did not know that the nurses were paid and that the type of service provided was difficult to price. She described a number of problems that were averted in terms of medication management, crisis management, recognition of problems at a stage where intervention prevented a medical problem, and helping people to find a physician when they had not already established such a relationship.

Another nurse had contracted with a congregate housing project whereby nursing care was prepaid along with rent. In one case, when a minimal fee-for-service stipulation was added, client utilization dropped to zero. The contractual arrangement was described as satisfactory for nursing. However, the nurse was then vulnerable to housing-management decisions regarding continuity of the service and choice of educational and pay level of the practitioner. Such a contract also meant that the nurse needed to facilitate patterns of usage in order not to miss people who needed the services, but perceived the nurse as too busy.

Another nurse has worked as an independent practitioner through contracts with a county and by offering nursing services in churches and in shopping centers. When she first started her practice, she wrote to doctors in order to generate referrals. One doctor referring a client reduced billing costs by 25 percent.

The county she contracts with pays her a flat rate of $15 per hour. She has "had no luck with Medicaid." She described the $15 per hour rate as satisfactory because she had little overhead except for her car, otoscope, sphygmomanometer, and blood glucose equipment.

The care she provides through the church is "free care." Some churches have requested blood pressure screenings without any in-depth counseling. Other churches have requested home care and nursing services in greater depth. She sees one benefit of her service in the opportunity to help others as she does not attend church regularly.

Another nurse, who owns community housing for the elderly, contracts for nursing services as part of the package. Nurses are paid $100 per month for supervising the health care of eight elderly residents. This pay includes two half-day visits per month to each house and response to phone calls residents or housing staff make to the nurses during the month. Nurses are paid $25 for assessments that are done prior to a resident's acceptance into the community housing. They are also paid additionally for workshops that they provide for housing staff.

Thus, a great variety of payment sources apart from third-party payments, were utilized by gerontological nurse specialists. However, payment for nursing services for the most part did not generate an income sufficient to live on and nurses either had to accept additional salaried positions, or were not the sole providers of financial support in their households.

Home Care

Two nurses were asked to describe their experiences regarding payment for home care nursing services. One nurse had started a home care agency and the other directed a proprietary agency. Because the regulations, number of agencies, and issues pertinent to home care alone would require a large study, data reported here are limited to a brief overview.

The nurse starting a new agency initially saw patients for free to generate the documentation necessary for obtaining a certificate of need and subsequent Medicare certification for psychiatric home care. Other insurance companies have also since paid for services of this agency. However, client needs usually were greater than the 40 visits customarily covered, so clients and their families then paid for care.

This respondent stated that she can no longer afford to accept clients with one major insurance company unless the clients agree to pay out of pocket. She described that company as being $20,000 behind in payments, and then only paying two percent per month.

Another nurse, who manages the metropolitan office of a nationwide proprietary home care agency, was also interviewed. This nurse reported that most of her clients paid with private insurance or out of pocket, although a few were covered by Medicare or Medicaid.

This respondent described home care as an area where many clients "fall through the cracks" in terms of having needs that Medicare does not cover, such as those who are not home-bound and may only need help with a bath. She described the $9 per-hour charge as more than what people on fixed incomes could afford to pay. Yet this rate was described as less than what nonproprietary agencies would charge for the same services.

The $20,000 in unpaid claims described by the first respondent was viewed as minor by this respondent in terms of that particular insurance company's overall unpaid claims. One HMO was described as covering home care services based on the nurses' assessment of client needs. However, this was not usually the case. Other HMOs were described as varying considerably in payment mechanisms. Services covered were described as not well defined, and were therefore dependent on the mood of the person with whom a home care agency happened to be dealing.

The experiences of home care nurses thus indicated that even when third-party payment was provided, collection of the payment was difficult, client needs exceeded the amount covered, and fees often exceeded clients' ability to pay. Coverage based on nursing assessment did occur, but most third-party payers required a physician order.

Nurse Generalists

Both nurse generalists interviewed were paid on a fee-for-service basis with a sliding scale based on ability to pay. Neither had been able to generate a profit above expenses. One practice ended after three years; another had been operating for six years.

In one case clients submitted their own claims for reimbursement and some were reimbursed by third-party payers. The other nurse interviewed had been reimbursed twice by a third-party payer and once by workmen's compensation benefits.

One nurse described her basic rates as $15 per hour for a workshop, $25 per hour for a hospital or home visit. She also had been paid $20 per hour as a nurse consultant for a physician group and had been paid through an agency for home health Title 18 visits.

The nurse generalists interviewed had found payments insufficient to support a practice financially. Problems in procuring third-party payment also were described by nurse generalists in that insurers did not recognize the services provided as payable services, such as outpatient counseling for post-partum depression or respite services for new patients or others caring for disabled persons.

SUMMARY

The respondents presented a picture of payment in Wisconsin that varied among specialty groups and among practitioners within each specialty group. Some nurses in each category had been paid directly, but this tended to be the exception rather than the rule.

Even when nurses were paid by third-party payers, client needs were reported as exceeding coverage, payments were difficult to collect, and in most specialty areas, payments received were insufficient for nurses to live on unless other sources of income were available. Records of client utilization, time spent, and types of service were kept by at least some members of each specialty group should such data be needed in further research.

POLICY ALTERNATIVES AND ANALYSIS

Based on the findings in this survey, it is evident that (1) the goal of strengthening nurses' control of nursing practice requires high priority, and (2) educational offerings dealing with payment issues are necessary across specialty groups so that payment sources utilized by some may be expanded to all areas of nursing practice. Additional attention to legislative changes mandating direct payment for nurses does not appear to be indicated at this time.

The caution against mandatory payment is based on the lack of support for mandatory payment and conclusion that the blocks to direct payment are largely perceptual and political on the part of insurers and HMOs identified by the Lakewood group (1985). Since third-party payments have been insufficient, difficult to collect, and inadequate in meeting clients' nursing-care needs even when nurses were included as providers, alternative sources of payment also need to be developed.

Boneparth (1982) described enhancement of equity as a value many would ascribe to making policy changes. Therefore changes in policy to increase direct payment of nurses would be best supported by evidence that such changes improve equity, but do not increase costs, decrease quality of care, or put other health care providers at risk of diminished tangible or intangible benefits.

The strongest case for equity would seem to be built by realizing (1) that 450,000 people in Wisconsin were uninsured (Reimer, 1984 cited in Murphy, 1986); (2) the usefulness of independent nursing practice as a means of addressing underserved populations (McKibbin, 1982); (3) the cost-effectiveness both for meeting the needs of underserved populations and decreasing overall health care costs, given that nurses are paid only one-third to one-fifth the amount physicians are paid for provision of identical services of equal or better quality (Aiken, Blendon, & Rogers, 1981; Jacox, 1984; U.S. Congress Office of Technology Assessment, 1986); and (4) the decreased client utilization of nurse providers whom insurers refused to pay (as supported by respondents in this study). The files of rejected insurance claims as well as records kept by nurses providing free nursing services identified by respondents in this study, also would support the case of inequity by identifying the need for independent nursing services and the current lack of payment.

Based on the findings of this study, it is recommended that nursing continuing education providers undertake the task of continuing education about direct payment issues. Invited papers reflecting data bases of nursing utilization and costs for clients could be distributed to conference participants and potential third-party payers.

Additional input for such a conference might be pursued by contacting businesses pursuing self-insurance mechanisms. These businesses also may be potential financial contributors to a conference exploring quality, cost-effective health care provision. Nurses can then use this information to better involve clients in pursuing direct payment as well as to inform employers, third-party payers, and legislators about options for quality, cost-effective health care.

REFERENCES

Aaronson, L. S. (1987). Nurse-midwives and obstetricians: Alternative models of care and client "Fit". *Research in Nursing and Health, 10,* 217–226.

Aiken, L. H. (Ed.) (1984). *Nursing in the 1980s crises, opportunities, challenges.* Philadelphia: J. B. Lippincott.

Aiken, L. H., Blendon R. J., & Rogers, D. E. (1981). The shortage of hospital nurses: A new perspective. *Annals of Internal Medicine, 95,* 365–372.

Alfano, G. J. (1982). Hospital-based extended care nursing: A case of study of the Loeb Center. In L. H. Aiken (Ed.), *Nursing in the 1980s crises, opportunities, challenges* (pp. 211–228). Philadelphia: J. B. Lippincott.

American Association of Nurse Anesthetists. (1986). *CRNA facts.* U.S. Congress: Office of Technology Assessment.

American Nurses' Association. (1984). *Obtaining third-party reimbursement: A position statement of the Commission on Economic and General Welfare.* Kansas City, MO: Author.

Bogdan, R. C., & Biklen, S. K. (1982). *Qualitative research for education: An introduction to theory and methods.* Boston: Allyn and Bacon, Inc.

Boneparth, E. (1982). A framework for policy analysis. In E. Boneparth (Ed.), *Women, power, and policy* (pp. 1–14). New York: Pergamon Press.

Brooten, D., Kumar, S., Brown, L., Butts, P., Finkler, S., Bakewell-Sachs, S., Gibbons, A., & Delivoria-Papdopoulos, M. (1986). A randomized clinical trial of early hospital discharge and home follow-up of very low birth weight infants. *New England Journal of Medicine, 315,* 934–939.

Bullough, B., Bullough, V. L., Garvey, J., & Allen, K. M. (1985). Third-party reimbursement for nurses. In B. Bullough, V. L. Bullough, J. Garvey, & K. M. Allen (Eds.), *Issues in nursing and annotated bibliography* (pp. 130–134). New York: Garland.

Gilbert, J. (1977). Outcome - experience and training of the anesthetist. In R. A. Hirsch (Ed.), *Health care delivery in anesthesia* (pp. 143–150). Philadelphia: George F. Stickly Co.

Harahan, M. (1987). *National long-term care channeling demonstration: Abstracts of reports.* Washington DC: Department of Health and Human Services.

Harrington, D., & Lempert, L. (1988). Medicaid: A public program in distress. *Nursing Outlook, 36,* 6–8.

Hartley, S., & McKibbin, R. C. (1983). *Economic and employment issues in nursing education.* Kansas City, MO: American Nurses' Association.

Jacox, A. K. (1984). Prospective payment: Focus on clinical nursing research. In C. A. Williams (Ed.), *Nursing research and policy formation: The case of prospective payment.* Kansas City, MO: American Academy of Nursing.

LaBar, C. (1983). *Third party reimbursement for services of nurses.* Kansas City, MO: American Nurses' Association.

LaBar, C. (1986). Legislation affecting the autonomy and credibility of nursing practice. *State Nursing Legislative Quarterly, 4*(1), 13–14.

Lakewood Group. (1985). *Analysis of reimbursement for nursing services in Wisconsin.* Madison, WI: The Wisconsin Nurses Association.

LeRoy, L. (1982). The cost effectiveness of nurse practitioners. In L. H. Aiken (Ed.), *Nursing in the 1980s crisis, opportunities, challenges* (pp. 295–314). Philadelphia: J. B. Lippincott.

Mayes, F., Oakley, D., Wranesh, B., Springer, N., Krumlauf, J., & Crosby, R. (1987). A retrospective comparison of certified nurse-midwife and physician management of low risk births. *Journal of Nurse-Midwifery, 32,* 216–221.

McKibbin, R. C. (1982). *Nursing in the '80s: Key economic and employment issues.* Kansas City, MO: American Nurses' Association.

Mullinax, K. (1987). Compliance with Medicaid reimbursement law as of November 1986. *Journal of Nurse-Midwifery, 32*(3), 159.

Murphy, E. K. (1986). Health care: Right or privilege. *Nursing Economics, 4*(2).

National League for Nursing. (1981). *Position statement on reimbursement for nursing care.* New York: National League for Nursing.

O'Malley, K. (1987). Nursing delivery systems that respond to emerging needs of special populations. *Post conference papers: National Commission on Nursing Implementation Project.* Milwaukee, WI: National Commission on Nursing.

Physician Payment Review Commission. (1988). *March 31, 1988 Report to Congress.* Washington DC: The Commission.

Poulin, M. A. (1985). *Configurations of nursing practice.* Kansas City, MO: American Nurses' Association.

Reimer, D. R. (1984). *Insuring Wisconsin's uninsured. Report submitted to the Wisconsin Department of Health and Social Services.* Madison, WI. November 12, 1984. Cited in Murphy (1986).

Roddy, P. C., & Hambelton, R. (1977). Supply, need and distribution of anesthesiologists and nurse anesthetists in the U.S. 1972 and 1980. *Medical Care, 15,* 750–766.

Spitzer, W. O. (1976). Evidence that justifies the introduction of new health professionals. In P. Slayton & M.J. Trebilcock (Eds.), *The professions and public policy* (pp. 211–236). Toronto: University of Toronto Press.

U.S. Congress Office of Technology Assessment (1986). *Nurse practitioners, physician assistants, and certified nurse-midwives: A policy analysis* (Health technology case study 37, OTA-HCS-37). Washington DC: US Government Printing Office.

Vogel, G. & Dolyesh, N. (1988). *Entrepreneuring: A nurse's guide to entrepreneuring and consulting.* New York: National League for Nursing.

5

Nursing Centers: State of the Art— Survey Results

Mary J. Roehrig, MSN, MA, RN

PURPOSE

The purpose of this survey was to ascertain commonalities in nursing centers related to eight major themes. These themes were:

1. Purpose
2. Organization
   a. staff
   b. consultants
3. Student clinical experience
   a. courses with clinical experience in center
   b. supervision of students
   c. evaluation of students
4. Services offered
5. Protocols established for services
6. Faculty practice criteria and role
7. Evaluation
   a. of services/nursing center

    b. of faculty
    c. of students
8. Quality assurance/audit system

"Nursing center" was the term used to describe a nurse-managed center. The coordinator/director was defined as the person primarily responsible for the daily management of the center.

PRECEDENTS IN LITERATURE

Frequently cited rationale for the development of nursing centers includes the provision of clinical experiences in primary care of the well client (Riesch, Felder, & Stauder, 1980); community service (Grimes & Stamps, 1980); faculty practice (Barger, 1986a, 1986b); and research facilitation (Ryan & Barger-Lux, 1985). Services often listed are history and physical examination (Culbert-Hinthorn, Fiscella, & Shortridge, 1985) and screening assessments (Hauf, 1977; Nettles-Carlson, Field, Friedman, & Smith, 1985); nutritional counseling (Ossler, Goodwin, Mariani, & Gilliss, 1982); educational programs (Arlton, 1986); and stress management (Baird & Benner, 1985).

    Though the positive student and faculty experiences have been well documented (Arlton, 1986; Culbert-Hindthorn, Fiscella, & Shortridge, 1985; Hauf, 1977; Ryan & Barger-Lux, 1985), standardization of protocol, policy, and procedures has been less clear. It appears that criteria for faculty practice and the role of faculty members practicing in the nursing center has been obscure for many fledgling nursing centers.

    Evaluation of client services (Bagwell, 1987), faculty practice, and student clinical experience are at an incipient stage. The need for a system of internal audit that is objective, flexible, and efficient is being sought by many nursing centers (Jones, 1976).

METHODOLOGY

To identify these commonalities, a survey requesting primarily yes/no responses to 10 questions related to the 8 major themes was sent to individuals associated with a nursing center or identified nursing centers. This survey appears on pages 75–77.

Sample

Eighty sample respondent names were selected from a list of participants at a nursing center seminar and respondents to another survey on nursing centers. This was the composite of both lists, and only those who were from the same center and students were eliminated. Of the 80, 3 were returned because of insufficient address data; 4 returned the questionnaire stating that either their clinic was closed or that they did not have a nursing center. Thus, the 30 remaining valid responses received were from a population of 73.

The 41 percent return rate did not include additional responses received after the 30 surveys were analyzed. Neither geographical area nor program differentiation (i.e., associate, baccalaureate, graduate) were eliminating factors. Returns were representative of each region in the United States. Though the type of program was not asked, it can be assumed from responses to course offerings and levels, and individual comments, that students were from baccalaureate or graduate programs.

DATA ANALYSIS

Because the purpose of the survey was simply to describe objective fact, it was necessary only to tally responses and convert them into percentages. For ease in comparison, percentages of yes answers based on n = 30 are presented in bar-graph form. To account for the questions and/or subquestions left unanswered, tables of percentages based on the actual number of respondents to the question are also included.

FINDINGS

Purpose

The most frequently listed purpose for a nursing center was to provide community service and education (90%); this was followed by student clinical experience (77%), research (70%), and faculty practice (57%). Other individual responses included institutional and student wellness, family planning, and a sexually transmitted disease clinic. Figure 1 illustrates this distribution.

Table 1 presents percentages based on the actual number of responses to that question.

Services

The most frequently listed services were physical assessment, client education, and counseling, followed by pap smear and lab tests. The graph in Figure 2 compares these five major categories along with the primary subcategories.

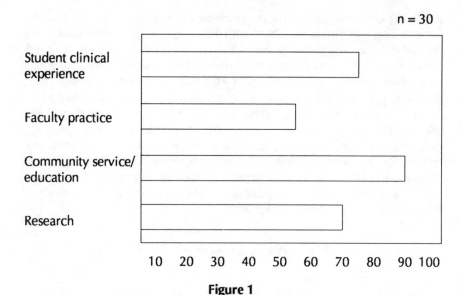

Figure 1
Purpose of Nursing Centers

Table 1
Purpose of Nursing Centers

Purpose	Percentage	Number of Responses
Student clinical experience	89	n = 26
Faculty practice	74	n = 23
Community service	96	n = 28
Research	81	n = 26

Tables 2–6 further differentiate services in each category. For comparison, the tables list percentages based on n = 30 and percentages based on the actual number of responses.

The question regarding client education focused on diabetes, hypertension, nutrition/weight control, stress management, and women's health issues. Additional topics listed by respondents included self-care responsibility, medication review, infant stimulation/parenting, fitness, substance control, sexually transmitted disease, child birth, smoking cessation, and "I Can Cope" (American Cancer Society) program.

Table 3 illustrates the breakdown of client education services.

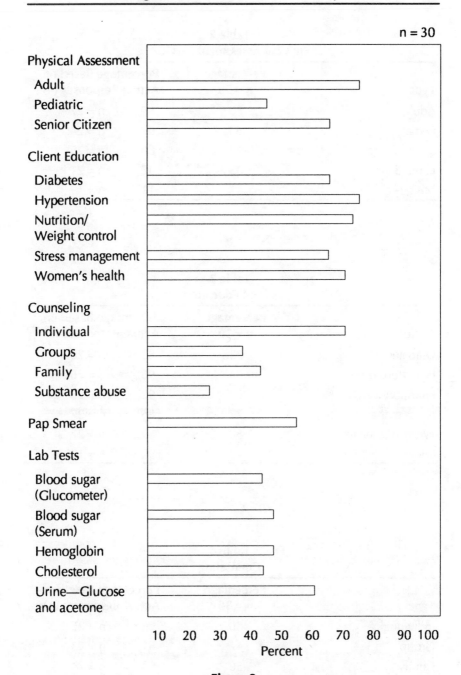

Figure 2
Services

Table 2
Physical Assessment Services

Type	Percentage n = 30	Percentage Based on Actual Responses (n)	
Adult	80	89	n = 27
Pediatric	53	67	n = 24
Senior citizen	73	88	n = 25
Limited	33	48	n = 21
Military	7	11	n = 19

Table 3
Client Education

Topic	Percentage n = 30	Percentage Based on Actual Responses (n)	
Diabetes	73	85	n = 26
Hypertension	83	96	n = 26
Nutrition/weight	80	92	n = 26
Stress management	77	85	n = 27
Women's health	80	89	n = 27
Other	40	92	n = 13

Table 4
Counseling

Type	Percentage n = 30	Percentage Based on Actual Responses (n)	
Individual	80	96	n = 25
Group	47	61	n = 23
Family	50	63	n = 24
Substance abuse	33	48	n = 21

Table 5
Lab Tests

Test	Percentage n = 30	Percentage Based on Actual Responses (n)	
Blood sugar—glucometer	67	71	n = 28
Blood sugar—serum	60	62	n = 29
Hemoglobin	60	64	n = 28
Blood typing	33	37	n = 27
Cholesterol	50	60	n = 25
SMAC	43	52	n = 25
VDRL	43	50	n = 26
Urine—glucose and acetone	70	75	n = 28
Other	27	73	n = 11

Individual, group, family, and substance-abuse counseling were reported; Table 4 illustrates the distribution of these responses.

Pap smears were performed by 63% of those surveyed or 70% of the 28 respondents who answered the question. Screening for communicable diseases and immunizations were services offered by 37% and 50%, respectively (n = 30). Table 5 lists the most frequently performed lab tests.

Other lab tests included pregnancy, strep, mononucleosis, electrolytes, hemoccults, and urine for protein, nitrites, and leukocytes; in fact it appeared that any lab test could be done if requested and ordered by a physician. Table 6 identifies the remaining services offered.

Developmental assessments, body mechanics, exercise, arthritis, pain management, BP monitoring, electrocardiogram, chest X-ray, and mammogram were services listed by individual respondents.

Table 6
Other Services

Service	Percentage n = 30	Percentage Based on Actual Responses (n)	
Foot care	60	72	n = 25
Ear irrigation	47	54	n = 26
Health risk appraisal	60	72	n = 25

Protocols

The second part of the service question asked for written protocols for services offered. Standing orders, U.S. Health Department, and state guidelines accounted for some protocols. "In process" or "being developed" explained four of the blank responses. This particular section of the survey was frequently left unanswered.

Tables 7–11 summarize the percentages of respondents who said they had written protocols for services.

Evaluation

The majority of nursing centers surveyed had some system of evaluation. Figure 3 compares methods of evaluation.

Physician Utilization (n = 30). Physicians provided direct services at a percentage rate of 27. Seventy percent of the nursing centers stated that they used a physician in a consultant capacity. Referrals comprised 60% by nursing centers and 47% of the respondents identified reliance on a physician for emergencies.

Contracts (n = 30). Written contracts for nursing center personnel/consultants numbered fewer than 50%; physicians, 37%; dietitian, 17%; staff nurse, 33%; faculty, 33%.

Supervision of Students (n = 30). Students were most frequently supervised by their instructor (47%). Full-time faculty practicing in the nursing center provided additional supervision (40%). Full-time staff nurses (30%), part-time faculty practicing in the nursing center (27%), and part-time staff nurses (13%) also supervised students.

Table 7
Protocols—Physical Assessment

Type	Percentage n = 30	Percentage Based on Actual Responses (n)	
Adult	37	58	n = 19
Pediatric	20	46	n = 13
Senior citizen	23	47	n = 15
Limited	10	25	n = 12
Military	3	11	n = 9

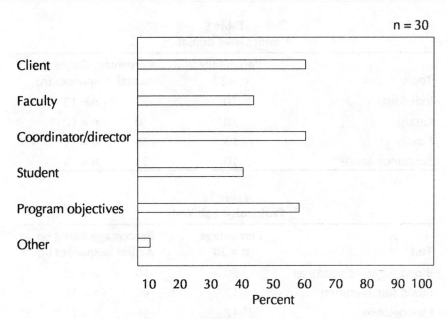

n = 30

Figure 3
Evaluation

Table 8
Protocols—Client Education

Topic	Percentage n = 30	Percentage Based on Actual Responses (n)	
Diabetes	27	50	n = 16
Hypertension	37	61	n = 18
Nutrition/weight	27	50	n = 16
Stress management	23	39	n = 18
Women's health	33	59	n = 17
Other	17	63	n = 8

Table 9
Protocols—Counseling

Topic	Percentage n = 30	Percentage Based on Actual Responses (n)	
Individual	10	23	n = 13
Group	10	30	n = 10
Family	13	36	n = 11
Substance abuse	10	33	n = 9

Table 10
Protocols—Lab Tests

Test	Percentage n = 30	Percentage Based on Actual Responses (n)	
Blood sugar—glucometer	20	50	n = 12
Blood sugar—serum	17	46	n = 11
Hemoglobin	17	46	n = 11
Blood typing	10	30	n = 10
Cholesterol	10	30	n = 10
SMAC	10	30	n = 10
VDRL	17	50	n = 10
Urine—glucose and acetone	20	55	n = 11
Other	13	50	n = 8

Table 11
Protocols—Other Services

Service	Percentage n = 30	Percentage Based on Actual Responses (n)	
Screen—Communicable disease	20	46	n = 13
Immunization	20	50	n = 12
Pap smear	27	67	n = 12
Foot care	17	42	n = 12
Ear irrigation	17	46	n = 11
Health risk appraisal	17	33	n = 15

Table 12
Criteria for Faculty Practice

Criterion	Percentage n = 30	Percentage Based on Actual Responses (n)	
Full-time appointment	33	59	n = 17
Part-time appointment	30	60	n = 15
Graduate degree	33	71	n = 14
ANA certification	13	27	n = 15
Physical assessment Verified by:			
course completion	27	62	n = 13
physician	3	11	n = 9
clinical nurse specialist	17	46	n = 11
other faculty member	3	14	n = 7

Criteria for Faculty Practice

Criteria for faculty practicing in the nursing center varied and frequently was left unanswered on the survey. This is summarized in Table 12.

Faculty Evaluation (n = 30). The method for evaluation of faculty members practicing in the nursing center also varied and likewise was frequently left unanswered. Thirty-three percent identified formal peer review, while 23% indicated informal peer review as a method of faculty evaluation. Client evaluation accounted for 17%, and the coordinator/director evaluated faculty in 33% of the cases.

Audit

Most respondents (70%, n = 30; 91%, n = 23) indicated that they had a system of chart audit. A quality assurance committee existed in 33% of the nursing centers (n = 30). A composite of membership included staff and community registered nurses, physician, social service counselor, dietitian, nursing faculty, senior baccalaureate and graduate students, certified nurse midwife, nursing administrators, non-nursing administrators, and accounting personnel.

Courses in which Clinical Experience Is Provided through the Nursing Center

The frequently listed course in which undergraduate nursing students received clinical experience in the nursing center was senior-level community health (11). Four respondents identified a senior practicum course (also called "Role Transition," "Independent Study," and "Professional Practice"). The remainder of undergraduate clinical courses included:

Med-Surg I	Freshman
Med-Surg Advanced	Senior
Nursing of children	Sophomore
Nursing of family	Junior
Health Assessment	Junior
Community Health	Junior
Nurse Process—Life span	Junior
Maternal–Child	Junior
Leadership	Senior
Management	Senior

Several graduate programs listed clinical experience in the nursing center. Among these were

Nurse midwifery

Nurse practitioner

Nurse practitioner—Pediatrics

Adult health

Community health

Primary care

Geriatric

Maternal–Child Health

Family primary care

Research teaching practicums were available to graduate students through the nursing center.

CONCLUSIONS

This survey set out to identify commonalities in nursing center purpose, management, and evaluation. Purpose appears to be the feature shared by most. Community service, student clinical experience, research, and faculty practice are the most frequently cited reasons for existence of the nursing center.

A similarity can also be seen in the type of services listed. Physical assessment, client education, and counseling are offered at the majority of nursing centers participating in the survey. Pap smear and certain lab tests, along with foot care and health risk appraisals are offered at more than half of the surveyed centers. The availability of written protocols was considerably less frequent, as were written contracts for nursing center personnel/consultants. Physician utilization was identified primarily for the purpose of consultation.

Students were most frequently supervised by their course instructor. Other faculty and nursing center staff provided supervision. Community health courses and senior-level practicums, along with graduate courses, were the predominating courses in which clinical experience in the nursing center was provided.

The criteria for the evaluation of faculty practice and method of evaluation leave much to speculation. Nearly half of the respondents left these two questions unanswered or only partially answered.

A system of chart audit was established in many nursing centers. A quality assurance committee functioned in several centers, and plans for such a committee were under way at others.

LIMITATIONS

Lack of consensus related to the conceptualization of nurse-managed nursing centers seems to be a problem inherent in researching an incipient organization. An academic definition of a nursing center (that is, a college- or university-operated center for the purpose of educational experiences and community service) versus a community definition as a nursing agency where students may go to receive clinical experience epitomizes such a lack of consensus. Until a clear definition has been established, data collection and subsequent analysis may lead to an equivocal conclusion.

Another limitation is the small sample size. It must be remembered, however, that the actual number of nursing centers is unknown but considered relatively small when compared to the number of nursing schools and nurses who could be providing independent nursing services.

Why respondents did not answer some or parts of the questions is also a concern.

RECOMMENDATIONS

An American Nurses' Association (ANA) task force is presently developing a definition of and guidelines for nurse-managed nursing centers. Full support is recommended for this effort. Collegial sharing is essential to the development of nursing centers of excellence. Dialogue and exchange of protocols, policies, procedures, research findings, and evaluations should be encouraged.

In this particular study, a review of the survey tool is recommended as well as follow-up letters to solicit additional returns for a delphi study.

REFERENCES

Arlton, D. (1986). A paying health promotion clinic: Combining client services and student learning. *Journal of Allied Health, 15*(1), 3–10.

Bagwell, M. (1987). Client satisfaction with nursing center services. *Journal of Community Health Nursing, 4*(1), 29–42.

Baird, S., & Benner, R. (1985). Keeping a university well with a health promotion clinic. *Nursing and Health Care, 6,* 97–100.

Barger, S. (1986a). Academic nurse-managed centers: Issue of implementation. *Family and Community Health, 9,* 12–22.

Barger, S. (1986b). Personnel issues in academic nurse-managed centers: The pitfalls and the potential. *Nurse Educator,* 11(3), 29–33.

Culbert-Hinthorn, P., Fiscella, K., & Shortridge, L. (1985). A nurse-managed clinical practice unit: Part 1—the positives. *Nursing and Health Care, 6*(2), 97–100.

Grimes, D., & Stamps, C. (1980). Meeting the health care needs of older adults through a community nursing center. *Nursing Administration Quarterly, 4*(3), 31–40.

Hauf, B. (1977). An evaluative study of a nursing center for community health nursing student experiences. *Journal of Nursing Education, 16*(8), 7–11.

Jones, A. (1976). Overview of a nursing center for family health services in Freeport. *Nurse Practitioner, 1*(6), 26–31.

Nettles-Carlson, B., Field, M., Friedman, B., & Smith, L. (1985). Group faculty practice: Dreams versus reality. *Nurse Educator, 10* (5), 8–12.

Ossler, C., Goodwin, M., Mariani, M., & Gilliss, C. (1982). Establishment of a nursing clinic for faculty and student clinical practice. *Nursing Outlook, 30*(7), 402–405.

Riesch, S., Felder, E., & Stauder, C. (1980). Nursing centers can promote health for individuals, families, and communities. *Nursing Administration Quarterly, 4*(3), 3–4.

Ryan, S. & Barger-Lux, J. (1985). Faculty expertise in practice: A school succeeding. *Nursing and Health Care, 6*(2), 75–78.

FERRIS STATE COLLEGE*

Department of Nursing

NURSING CENTER SURVEY

In this questionnaire, the terms "Nursing Center" and "Coordinator/Director" are used respectively to describe a nurse-managed center and the person who has primary responsibility for the daily management of the Center.

1. What is the purpose of your Nursing Center?

	NO	YES
Student clinical experience?	___	___
Faculty practice?	___	___
Community service/education?	___	___
Research of Nursing problems?	___	___
Other? (please explain)	___	___

2. What services do you offer? Do you have written protocols for these services?

	Services		Protocols	
	NO	YES	NO	YES**
Physical Assessment				
Adult?	___	___	___	___
Pediatric?	___	___	___	___
Senior Citizen?	___	___	___	___
Limited (Sports, School)?	___	___	___	___
Military?	___	___	___	___
Client Education				
Diabetes?	___	___	___	___
Hypertension?	___	___	___	___
Nutrition/Weight Control?	___	___	___	___
Stress Management?	___	___	___	___
Women's Health Issues?	___	___	___	___
Other? (please list)	___	___	___	___
Screening for Communicable Disease?	___	___	___	___
Immunizations?	___	___	___	___
Pap Smear?	___	___	___	___
Ear Irrigation?	___	___	___	___
Lab procedures				
Blood sugar with glucometer?	___	___	___	___
Serum blood sugar?	___	___	___	___
Hemoglobin?	___	___	___	___
Blood typing?	___	___	___	___
Cholesterol?	___	___	___	___
SMAC or Chemistry Profile?	___	___	___	___
VDRL?	___	___	___	___
Urine for glucose & acetone?	___	___	___	___
Other? (please list)	___	___	___	___

*Ferris State College has since achieved university status
**If you have written protocols and would be willing to exchange them, please indicate on enclosed postcard.

	Services		Protocols	
	NO	YES	NO	YES**
Health Risk Appraisal?	___	___	___	___
Counseling				
Individual?	___	___	___	___
Group?	___	___	___	___
Family?	___	___	___	___
Substance Abuse?	___	___	___	___

3. How are services evaluated?

	NO	YES
Client survey?	___	___
Faculty evaluation?	___	___
Coordinator/Director evaluation?	___	___
Student evaluations?	___	___
Program objectives?	___	___
Other? (please explain)	___	___

4. Do you have a physician available on staff?

For direct client services?	___	___
As a consultant?	___	___
For referrals?	___	___
In emergency situations?	___	___

5. Do you have written contracts for specific assignments in the Nursing Center?

Physician?	___	___
Dietician?	___	___
Staff Nurses (non-faculty)?	___	___
Faculty?	___	___

6. What courses have a clinical component or lab scheduled in the Nursing Center? Please list the course name and level of student.

COURSE   LEVEL OF STUDENT

7. Who supervises student clinical experiences in the Nursing Center?

	NO	YES
Instructor of course?	___	___
Full-time faculty practicing in the Nursing Center?	___	___
Part-time faculty practicing in the Nursing Center?	___	___
Full-time staff nurse?	___	___
Part-time staff nurse?	___	___

8. Criteria for faculty practice include:

	NO	YES
Full-time faculty appointment?	___	___
Part-time faculty appointment?	___	___
Graduate degree?	___	___
ANA Certification in Clinical Specialty?	___	___
If yes, do faculty practice in specialty area?	___	___

Demonstration of physical assessment skills verified by:

	NO	YES	If yes, how often?
Completion of physical assessment course?	___	___	_____
Physician?	___	___	_____
Clinical Nurse Specialist (certified)?	___	___	_____
Another faculty member?	___	___	_____
Other? (please list)	___	___	_____

9. What mechanisms are used for faculty evaluation?

	NO	YES
Formal peer review?	___	___
Informal peer review?	___	___
Client evaluations?	___	___
Coordinator/Director evaluation?	___	___
Other? (please describe)	___	___

10. What system for chart auditing is useful in your agency?

Checklist for completion of forms	___	___
Quality assurance committee	___	___

If you have a quality assurance committee, what are the disciplines/backgrounds of people on the committee?

Please return questionnaire in the envelope provided. Thank you.

6

Assessing the Effects of Clinical Setting on Students' Attitudes Toward Professional Autonomy and Client Advocacy

Jo A. Brooks, DNS, RN, C
Paul Femea, DNSc, RN

Achievement of autonomy is a major step in nursing's struggle for full professional status. Mundinger (1980) asserts that autonomy is a necessary attribute of professional practice. Much of the socialization into the professional role occurs during the educational process. Therefore, it is incumbent on nurse educators to examine curriculum and educational experiences to ensure that they inculcate those attitudes and values that are essential for professional nursing.

Some have suggested that schools of nursing tend to discourage or limit autonomy in students. Leininger (1970) and Cohen (1981) identify the regimentation of students and the rigid educational experiences as problems that fail to support the development of professional autonomy among students. Others have studied the characteristics of students who choose nursing and suggested that those students do not possess characteristics that reflect an autonomous nature (Boughn, 1988).

As a faculty in a baccalaureate program we have identified that one of our goals is to prepare a graduate who will value professional autonomy and respect the rights of clients/patients to be informed about and participate in their own care.

PURPOSE

The purpose of this study is (1) to determine if there is any difference in attitudes toward autonomy, patient rights, and traditional nursing roles among entering generic nursing students, students at the completion of the baccalaureate program, and upper-division of registered nurse students; and (2) to determine if the clinical setting influences the attitudes and values of these students.

BACKGROUND

This study is a continuation of a study we conducted as a part of the evaluation of the Division of Nursing grant we received to develop the Nursing Center for Family Health (NCFH). At that time (January 1, 1981–December 31, 1983), the Purdue University School of Nursing offered an upper-division baccalaureate program. As the objectives for the NCFH were developed we believed that such a learning experience would produce a student who recognizes that professional nursing has autonomous functions, who believes that clients are responsible for their own health, and who questions the limitations of the traditional role as it relates to the practice of professional nursing.

We utilized the Pankratz Nursing Questionnaire (PNQ) which was developed in 1974 to measure aspects of professional autonomy and advocacy in nursing. The questionnaire grew from the authors' concern that autonomy, which was defined as independence of practice, was not being fostered in basic nursing programs. Dependence versus independence was considered from three perspectives: (1) dependence versus independence for the nurse called "nursing autonomy", (2) dependence versus independence for the patient ("patient rights"), and (3) rejection of traditional nursing role limitations.

Using a repeated measure design in the original study, we found that students who had a 15-week clinical experience either in public health nursing or in the leadership and management course in the NCFH had greater increases in all three of the subscales. There were also significant differences in the mean scores on the three subscales of those students who had a clinical experience in the NCFH.

In 1980 the school of nursing made the decision to move to a four-year generic program. The first class was admitted in August 1982. This was the second year of the grant and as we collected data at the end of the academic year for the evaluation of the grant, we discussed whether this was a study we wanted to continue as we moved into the generic curriculum. The subcommittee on program evaluation felt it would fit into the overall evaluation plan and recommended that we continue the study at the completion of the grant.

METHODOLOGY

Starting in the fall of 1985, the PNQ was administered to entering freshmen as part of a battery of pre-post measures that are variables in our curriculum plan. We have now collected data on incoming students in Fall 1985, 1986, and 1987. One hundred-eighty-seven usable questionnaires were returned. Originally, our plan was to replicate the repeated measure design utilized in the evaluation of the grant for the NCFH. Each class would be given the PNQ at the completion of the generic program. When we realized that it would be 1990 before we would have an adequate sample, we changed the design of the study because our student body is a homogeneous group—basically white, female, age 18–21—we decided to implement a correlated-group design. We administered the PNQ to the first graduating class in May 1986, again as part of the curriculum evaluation plan, and to each succeeding senior class. We now have data on 237 graduating seniors.

Instrument

In a research study completed in 1974, Loren and Deanna Pankratz focused on the views of nurses regarding dependence versus independence for both nurses and patients. They wished to study the level of autonomy of nurses with different levels of education in various settings, since autonomy is regarded as an essential component of professionalism. The research was divided into two dimensions: nursing autonomy and patients' rights. The first refers to the nurse's perception of how much latitude nurses have or are willing to take in functioning as responsible professionals. The latter dimension focuses on patients' present and allowed range of knowledge about their own care and their participation in the same.

A 69-item questionnaire was constructed and administered to 200 RNs in a large community hospital. Preliminary results indicated that the factors of interest were present and encouraged further presentation of the form to other nurses. Two community hospitals, two university hospitals, and a large psychiatric hospital were selected in order to provide diverse sampling of nurses. In addition to the subjects obtained from these three facilities, 206 nursing administrators were also included in the study, providing a total of 702 subjects.

A principal component factor analysis resulted in three subscales that adequately represented the intent of the study: (1) nursing autonomy and advocacy, (2) patients' rights, and (3) rejection of traditional role limitations. Pankratz and Pankratz (1974) defined each of these variables as follows:

1. Nursing autonomy and advocacy are defined as the extent to which nurses feel comfortable in taking initiative and responsibility in the hospital.
2. Patients' rights are defined as the nurse's hypothetical concession of certain rights to patients.
3. Rejection of traditional role limitations is defined as the nurse's willingness to openly disagree with the doctor and to become highly involved in the personal matters of patients.

The subscales clearly differentiated between the different samples of nurses. Higher scores were associated with education, leadership, academic setting, and nontraditional social climate.

The authors of the tool indicate that the study provides no information regarding the reliability of the instrument, although it has been used since. Murray and Morris (1982) utilized the PNQ in a study of autonomy in three different nursing education programs but did not provide any information regarding reliability.

We did find that we had a small group of seniors (N = 30) who inadvertently responded to the questionnaire two times within the week the PNQ was administered in senior nursing courses. We found the means in the three subscales for this paired sample did not differ significantly (p = .001), and therefore we feel the students answers were consistent.

Scoring the Instrument. A 5-point Likert scale is used where "1" equals "strongly agree," "2" equals "agree," "3" equals "undecided," "4" equals "disagree," and "5" equals "strongly disagree." The subscales are scored using a system developed by Tryon and Bailey. For the nursing autonomy subscale the possible range is 70–130, with the most autonomous nurse having the highest score. The range for patient rights is 14–70; a nurse who recognizes that patients have rights would score higher than a nurse who denies patients rights. The scores on rejection of traditional role limitations (role) can range from a low of 12 to a high of 60. Those scoring low reflect what Haberstein and Christ (1955) first categorized as "traditionalizers," nurses whose primary loyalty is to patients and see themselves as subordinate to physicians, while those who score high would be categorized as "professionalizer."

LIMITATIONS

The limitations of this study include the following: (1) It is not possible to control all variables within the clinical setting and their effects on students' attitudes. Students may have a wide variety of experiences because of client scheduling quirks, time of semester, and the faculty who supervised their clinical experience; (2) The validity of measuring attitudes through written responses to questions, and then arbitrarily quantifying the answers has been questioned by many researchers. The degree that the data measure the respondents' true attitudes depends on how honest they were when answering the questions. For this group we do have limited evidence that the students did answer truthfully. Thirty students took the PNQ twice within the same posttest period and their mean scores were essentially identical, indicating that they answered consistently on both tests; (3) Shatzenhafer (1987) points out that although the PNQ has been used for more than a decade to measure autonomy it actually measures three interrelated variables: nurse autonomy, patient rights, and rejection of the traditional nursing role. Schatzenhafer states that several items concurrently measure two variables and several items are ambiguously worded; (4) Student participation in the evaluation is confidential and voluntary. Therefore, we do not always get 100% participation. The percentage of students completing the PNQ has varied from a high of 84% in 1987 to a low of 55% in 1988.

DATA ANALYSIS

Preliminary analysis indicates that there were significant differences in students' scores on the three subscales on the PNQ between entering freshmen and graduating seniors, with seniors having higher means than freshmen. We wondered if these seniors in the generic baccalaureate were different from the RN seniors in the upper-division baccalaureate program we had previously studied. We decided to add the RN group so that we would have three levels of students: generic freshmen, seniors, and upper-division seniors. As we expected, there were still significant differences. Freshmen in the generic program scored lower than graduating seniors in the same program, who, in turn, scored lower than the RN students in the upper-division program on autonomy, rights, and role. The range of scores of the students on the scales were: autonomy, 54–124; rights, 46–70; and role, 18–60. Table 1 shows the means and results of analysis of variance for the differences in means among the three levels of students for the three subscales of the PNQ.

There was a positive significant relationship (p=<.05) between age and the three subscales. The strongest relationship was between age and autonomy, which had a correlation of 0.37, and the lowest correlation was between age and rights (r=0.21). When we examined experience we found there was a positive nonsignificant relationship between the three subscales among the three levels of students. The strongest relationship was between experience and autonomy (r=0.61), followed by experience and rights with a correlation of 0.57, and experience and roles (r=0.41).

In the original study, placement in the NCFH for clinical experience was a significant variable, but it demonstrated no effect on the scores of the graduating seniors in the generic program on any of the subscales.

DISCUSSION

It is apparent from the data analysis that the students in the generic baccalaureate program become more autonomous as they progress through the curriculum. They make their greatest gains in the autonomy subscale. We would anticipate that within five years their scores would be no different than the RN group. This would seem to provide credence to Cohen's theory of professional development in which she identifies four stages of professional development. According to Cohen (1981) nurses leave their educational program at Stage III–Mutuality, and after a period of experience achieve Stage IV–Interdependence, or internalized professionalism.

The entering freshmen come into the program recognizing the concept of patient rights. Their scores are not significantly different from the pretest scores of the RN students in the old upper-division program. This may reflect the growing public awareness and acceptance of the concept of patient rights. Although the differences between the three levels of students are significant, the gains in the mean scores are very low.

Beginning freshmen do not have a clear idea of what the role of the professional nurse is they become socialized in the role during their educational program, their conception of the role becomes more professional. This is reflected in the change in scores on roles of freshmen to graduating seniors. One of our most puzzling findings, in view of our previous study, is that placement in the NCFH had no effect and may even have had a negative effect on the graduating seniors' scores on all three of the subscales of the PNQ. One possible explanation could be the timing of the administration of the questionnaire. If a student had a clinical experience in the NCFH in the fall semester, that student would have responded to the questions four months

Table 1
Summary of Results of the Analysis

I. Comparison of Mean Scores

	Autonomy	Patients' Rights	Rejection of Traditional Role
Freshmen	77.66	58.46	41.17
Generic seniors	92.48	61.03	47.89
Upper-division	94.39	60.03	48.31

II. Anaylsis of Variance

	Autonomy		Patients' Rights		Rejection of Traditional Role	
	F-ratio	Probability	F-ratio	Probability	F-ratio	Probability
Age	13.891	0.00	2.717	0.0019	10.084	0.00
Level	15.868	0.00	15.868	0.00	139.323	0.00
Experience	5.684	0.00	3.121	0.0054	3.495	0.0023
Course	1.837	0.1420	3.579	0.015	0.874	0.4558

later, at the end of a semester in which the clinical experiences are primarily in traditional acute-care settings. In the study conducted with RN students during the grant period the PNQ was administered during the students' last clinical days in the NCFH. If this is true, then the effect of clinical setting would not appear to be as long lasting as we had hoped.

A second possible explanation also related to timing is the fact that we ask faculty to administer this battery of evaluation tools at the end of the semester, at the same time faculty and students must complete several other tasks. Students may feel they are tested too much and refuse to complete the questionnaire. Some faculty may not value the importance of evaluation and their attitude may influence the students' response rate. Since the responses are confidential and voluntary, it is impossible to follow up with nonrespondents.

We did find the response rate varied from a high of 84% for the class of 1987, to a low of 55% for the class of 1988. Among the 23 students who were in the NCFH in Spring 1988, only 29% completed the questionnaire. This small N does not allow satisfactory comparisons. Perhaps these students manifest autonomy by not responding.

The results of this study are very similar to those reported by Murray and Morris (1982). Our graduating seniors had mean scores on autonomy and patient rights that were quite similar to those in the baccalaureate program studied by Murray and Morris. It would appear that our curriculum does promote autonomy. The mean scores on rejection of traditional roles are lower for our graduating seniors than Murray and Morris presented. We need to examine the factors that may influence students' attitudes toward the nurse's role, and implement strategies to strengthen their conception of the professional role. To test the hypothesis that graduates' scores on autonomy will continue to increase after leaving the baccalaureate program, we need to add the PNQ to our graduate follow-up questionnaire.

REFERENCES

Boughn, S. (1988). A lack of autonomy in the contemporary nursing student: A comparative study. *Journal of Nursing Education, 27,* 150–155.

Cohen, H. (1981). *The nurse's quest for a professional identity.* Menlo Park, CA: Addison-Wesley Publishing.

Haberstein, R.W., & Christ, E.A. (1985). *Professionalizer, traditionalizer and utilizer.* Columbia, MO: University of Missouri.

Leininger, M.M. (1970). *Nursing and anthropology: Two worlds to blend.* New York: Wiley.

Mundinger, M. (1980). *Autonomy in nursing.* Maryland: Aspen Systems Corp.

Murray, L.M., & Morris, D.R. (1982). Professional autonomy among senior nursing students in diploma, associate degree and baccalaureate nursing programs. *Nursing Research. 31*, 311–313.

Pankratz, L., & Pankratz, D. (1974). Nursing autonomy and patient rights: Development of a nursing attitude scale. *Journal of Health and Social Behavior, 56*, 211–216.

Schatzenhafer, K.K. (1987). The measurement of professional autonomy. *Journal of Professional Nursing, 3*, 278–283.

Tryon, R.C., & Bailey, D.E. (1966). The B.C. Try computer system of cluster and factor analysis. *Multivariate Behavioral Research, 1*, 95–111.

BIBLIOGRAPHY

Betz, C.L. (1985). Students in transition: Imitators of role models. *Journal of Nursing Education, 24*, 301–303.

Botherton, S.E. (1988). Nursing role orientation of three groups: From naive to realistic. *Journal of Nursing Education, 27*, 117–123.

Boughn, S. (1988). A lack of autonomy in the contemporary nursing student: A comparative study. *Journal of Nursing Education, 27*, 150–155.

Cohen, H. (1981). *The nurse's quest for a professional identity.* Menlo Park, CA: Addison-Wesley Publishing.

Goldstein, J. (1980). Comparison of graduating AD and baccalaureate nursing students' characteristics. *Nursing Research, 29*, 45–48.

Haberstein, R.W., & Christ, E.A. (1985). *Professionalizer, traditionalizer and utilizer.* Columbia, MO: University of Missouri.

Itano, J.K., Warren, J.J., & Ishida, L.N. (1987). A comparison of role conceptions and role deprivation in baccalaureate students in nursing participating in a preceptorship or a traditional clinical program. *Journal of Nursing Education, 26*, 69–73.

Murray, L.M., & Morris, D.R. (1982). Professional autonomy among senior nursing students in diploma, associate degree and baccalaureate nursing programs. *Nursing Research, 31*, 311–313.

Pankratz, L., & Pankratz, D. (1974). Nursing autonomy and patient rights: Development of a nursing attitude scale. *Journal of Health and Social Behavior, 15*, 211–216.

Schatzenhafer, K.K. (1987). The measurement of professional autonomy. *Journal of Professional Nursing, 3*, 278–283.

Singleton, E.K., & Nail, F.C. (1984). Autonomy in nursing. *Nursing Forum, 21*, 123–130.

7

An Epidemiological Study of Hypercholesterolemia in a University Community

Jo A. Brooks, DNS, RN, C
Paul Femea, DNSc, RN

One of the ongoing programs offered each fall by the Nursing Center for Family Health (NCFH) since its opening in 1981 is its campus-wide blood pressure screening program. The screening has served as an excellent case-finding strategy and provides the center with increased visibility. In the fall of 1988 we decided to forego blood-pressure screening and offer a campus-wide cholesterol screening program. A large body of epidemiological evidence supports a direct relationship between increased blood cholesterol levels and an increased risk of coronary heart disease (CHD). Risk of CHD rises proportionately with cholesterol level, particularly when cholesterol levels rise above 200 mg/dl (Lipid Research Clinics Program, 1984a,b). In view of the media attention being paid to cholesterol and the recommendations coming from the surgeon general's office that all adults over the age of 20 should have their cholesterol level checked, we felt that this program would have wide appeal.

Several prospective studies have shown consistently that serum cholesterol levels predict the future occurrence of CHD morbidity and mortality (Martin, Hulley, Browner, Kuller, & Wentworth, 1986), therefore, we felt this was a program that would be of great benefit to the university students and young faculty and staff alike. If we could identify young adults (19–34) who had cholesterol levels that exceeded the "desirable blood cholesterol levels" identified by the 1987 National Cholesterol Education Program Adult Treatment Panel, we could intervene with dietary therapy. The goal of such therapy is to reduce the number of individuals with high-risk low-density lipoprotein (LDL) levels of cholesterol to levels below 160 mg/dl, the cutoff point for initiating drug therapy. Each 1% reduction in serum cholesterol yields approximately a 2% reduction in CHD rates.

Because most of the cholesterol in the serum is found in LDL, the concentration of total cholesterol is closely correlated with the concentration of LDL-cholesterol. Thus a total cholesterol that does not require fasting can be used in the initial stage of evolution.

Our interest in cholesterol screening was heightened upon reviewing the results of a successful program carried out in Marion County, Indiana in April 1987. The program was sponsored by a local television station, the Marion County Heart Association, and Boehringer Mannheim, the manufacturer of the Reflotron®, a device for measuring serum cholesterol levels. After making contact with the manufacturer and viewing an on-site demonstration, we felt this was a service which fit into the long-range goals of the NCFH.

The availability of a portable dry-blood analyzer that allows testing with capillary blood (permitting sampling from a finger prick rather than a venipuncture) makes it logistically and economically feasible to offer mass cholesterol screenings. Boehringer Mannheim Diagnostics (BMD) Division has supported community cholesterol programs through their loan purchase program, and advertises extensively in the *American Journal of Public Health*. BMD provides not-for-profit community agencies an opportunity to offer cholesterol screening and generate money to purchase a Reflotron®. For each BMD Reflotron® purchased, the company will loan 4 units for up to 10 days. The Reflotron® has been widely used for such large scale programs and has a reported reliability of .98.

We were interested in collecting data on a young adult population in terms of cholesterol levels and the presence of identified risk factors. Our experience with blood pressure screening indicated that, although this population attained higher levels of education, it reflected the blood pressure norms reported for this age group from the National Institute of Health. Therefore, we anticipated that cholesterol levels would reflect the prevalence of high blood cholesterol in the United States as reported by the National Center for Health Statistics in 1986. Based on those data, we expect to find 10.5% of white males and 9.45% of white females age 19–35 to have total cholesterol levels ≥ 200 mg/dl.

METHODS

Screening took place at Stewart Center and at the School of Nursing, Purdue

University. The university has 33,000 students and 7,747 faculty and staff at the West Lafayette campus. These two sites were selected so that a maximal number of people would be within a 10-minute walk to either site. As only total cholesterol was being measured, fasting samples were not required for the screening. Because we had an agreement to purchase one Reflotron® the company loaned us four units for the two-week screening program; this allowed us to operate five screening stations.

Screening Procedures

Screenings were held 9 a.m. – 2 p.m., Monday through Friday for two weeks in the fall semester. The program was staffed by nursing faculty and students enrolled in senior nursing courses. The business office provided a person to collect fees at the Stewart Center site and the secretary of the NCFH collected fees at the School of Nursing site. The fee for the screening was set at $3.00. This fee covered the cost of supplies plus $1.20 per test toward the purchase of the Reflotron®.

Since the Stewart Center site was close to the center of the campus, we placed three blood analyzers there. This required a staff of eight: one check-in person, two persons to perform finger sticks, three to operate blood analyzers, and two for debriefing. At the School of Nursing site we operated two blood analyzers with a staff of six or seven persons: one to check in and collect fees, two to perform finger sticks, two to run blood analyzers, and one to do debrief. The screening sites were set up as follows:

Check-in. After paying the $3 fee, each participant filled out a cholesterol screening card (Figure 1). The card asked for demographic data and contained a series of questions related to lifestyle, diet, health history, and family health history, and included a statement of consent with a place for the participant's signature. The questions were generated from the variables identified in the Multiple Risk Factor Intervention Trial (Stamler, Wentworth, & Neaton, 1986) and the report of the 1984 Consensus Development Conference on Lowering Blood Cholesterol to Prevent Heart Disease.

Finger sticks*. After completing the screening card, participants moved to the finger sticking station as openings became available. The screening card was checked for signature and then each participant had his or her finger cleansed with an alcohol swab, dried with a 2x2 gauze square, and pricked with a lancet; 30 microliters (0.03 ml.) of blood was drawn into a lithium-heparinized capillary tube. Occasionally air would enter the tube and a second tube would be needed to obtain an adequate sample.

---

*Nursing students and faculty performing finger sticks and operating the blood analyzer utilized universal precautions as specified by CDC.

Location _____   NCFH (1) _____

Identification No. _____   AWS (2) _____

Initial Screening Date ___/___/___   Other (3) _____

Name _____ Telephone No. (___) ___-___

Local Address _____ ZIP _____

Social Security Number ___-___-___ (optional)

Birth Date ___/___/___ Sex: M ___ (1) F ___ (2) Race: Caucasian ___ (1) Black ___ (2) Other ___ (3) (specify) _____

Height _____ Weight _____ Frame: Small _____ Medium _____ Large _____

Marital Status: Single (1) _____ Married (2) _____ Widowed (3) _____ Divorced (4) _____

Student _____ (1) Staff _____ (2) Other _____ (9) Highest Grade Completed _____ (years)

(Please turn the card over and complete.)

                #1   #2   #3

Total Blood Cholesterol Results _____ mg/dl _____ mg/dl _____ mg/dl

              See instructions below

1. Record the initial test result in #1.
2. If the initial test result is greater than 300 mg/dL or less than 100 mg/dL, do a second test and enter the result in #2. If this second determination confirms the first result (i.e., within ±5%), it is not necessary to do any further testing.
3. If the second determination does not confirm the first result (i.e., varies by more than ±5%), do a third test, and enter the result in #3.

                              Nurse's Signature _____

I hereby release the Nursing Center for Family Health, School of Nursing, Purdue University and all persons connected with them and any other organization associated with this screening, from any and all liability arising from or in any way connected to blood drawing for my blood cholesterol measurement or from the data derived therefrom.

                              Signature _____

Figure 1

Top: Serum Cholesterol Screening: Participant Data; Blood Cholesterol Result Data; Consent and Release Statement; Bottom: Lifestyle Questions.

Lifestyle Questions

1. Do you smoke tobacco? _____ Yes _____ No
2. If answer is yes, how much do you smoke per day? _____ 2 packs of cigarettes or more. _____ 1 1/2–2 packs of cigarettes. _____ 1 1/2 packs of cigarettes. _____ 1/2–1 pack of cigarettes. _____ less than 1/2 pack of cigarettes or light pipe or cigar.
3. How many years have you smoked?
4. Are you a former smoker? _____ 5. How long ago did you quit?
6. How often do you feel anxious or stressed? _____ Rarely _____ Sometimes _____ Often Do you find it difficult to relax? _____ Yes _____ No _____ Sometimes
7. Do you do at least 20 minutes of vigorous conditioning exercise? _____ 3 times a week _____ less than 3 times a week _____ not at all
8. Which single answer best describes your daily activity? _____ a lot (extra heavy labor) _____ some (extra housework) _____ very little (desk)
9. How often do you consume:

lean ham, beef, lamb	_____ rarely/never	_____ 1–2 times/wk	_____ 3–4 times/wk	_____ 5 or more/wk
eggs	_____ rarely/never	_____ 1–2 times/wk	_____ 3–4 times/wk	_____ 5 or more/wk
liver (chicken, beef)	_____ rarely/never	_____ 1–2 times/wk	_____ 3–4 times/wk	_____ 5 or more/wk
sardines, oil packed	_____ rarely/never	_____ 1–2 times/wk	_____ 3–4 times/wk	_____ 5 or more/wk
butter	_____ rarely/never	_____ 1–2 times/wk	_____ 3–4 times/wk	_____ 5 or more/wk
Canadian bacon	_____ rarely/never	_____ 1–2 times/wk	_____ 3–4 times/wk	_____ 5 or more/wk
lobster/shrimp	_____ rarely/never	_____ 1–2 times/wk	_____ 3–4 times/wk	_____ 5 or more/wk

Your Health History

Do you have any of the following? 1. Coronary artery disease _____ Yes _____ No 2. High blood pressure _____ Yes _____ No
3. Diabetes _____ Yes _____ No 4. High cholesterol level _____ Yes _____ No
Are you currently taking: Birth control pills _____ Yes _____ No Estrogen _____ Yes _____ No

Family Health History

Do you know if a *blood relative* has had any of the following diseases? 1. Heart attack before age 50 _____ Yes _____ No
2. Stroke before age 50 _____ Yes _____ No 3. High blood pressure _____ Yes _____ No 4. Diabetes _____ Yes _____ No
5. High cholesterol level _____ Yes _____ No 6. Coronary artery disease _____ Yes _____ No

Figure 1

Top: Serum Cholesterol Screening; Participant Data; Blood Cholesterol Result Data; Consent and Release Statement; Bottom: Lifestyle Questions.

Blood analyzer*. The participant carried his or her capillary tube and screening card to the operator of the blood analyzer. The operator of the analyzer transferred the blood sample to the testing strip. A sample can remain in the capillary tube for up to 6 minutes but must be inserted in the blood analyzer within 15 seconds after transferring it to testing strip; the operator had to remain aware of time and alert finger stickers to delay if analysis was running behind. The analyzer needs approximately 173 seconds to complete the analysis and obtain readings. If the operator had one sample in the machine and one capillary tube waiting, the finger stickers would have to delay. While waiting, the operator reviewed the cholesterol screening card to make sure the participant had answered all the questions and discuss any answers that indicated the risk of CHD. Although the Reflotron® is capable of processing 20 samples per hour, we found that if we took more than 14 samples per hour, we had to delay participants because of the teaching that took place at every station.

When the results appeared on the digital readout, the operator gave the participant a slip of paper with the results and a brief statement indicating either a normal or elevated reading; the participant was then directed to the debriefing station.

Debriefing. At this station a nursing student or faculty member reviewed the participant's results. Using the criteria developed by the Expert Panel on the Detection, Evaluation and Treatment of High Blood Cholesterol in Adults (Table 1), recommendations for follow-up were made. A variety of educational materials were available.

RESULTS

Demographics

A total of 938 participants were screened among whom 888 had usable data recorded on their cholesterol screening cards. Of the 888, 50.8% were male and 49.2% were female. Approximately 97% were white and 3% were nonwhite. The mean cholesterol level (MCL) for the total population was 182.5 mg/dl. Forty-four percent of the group were between the ages of 19 and 35; 36.2% were students, 50% were faculty and staff, and 13.8% were either visitors who happened to be on campus that day or family of students or faculty and staff who came to campus to get their cholesterol levels checked.

Sixty percent were single, 36.3% were married, and 3.3% divorced or widowed. The educational level for the group reflects the kind of community

---

*Nursing students and faculty performing finger sticks and operating the blood analyzer utilized universal precautions as specified by CDC.

Table 1
Recommendations for Follow-up

Total Cholesterol < 200 mg/dl	Repeat within 5 years
	Provide general dietary and risk factor education
Total Cholesterol 200–239 mg/dl	Provide information on Step 1 diet
Without definite CHD or two risk factors	Repeat cholesterol measurement annually
With definite CHD or two risk factors	Remeasure total cholesterol in 1 month
	Reinforce dietary education
Total Cholesterol > 240 mg/dl	Lipoprotein Analysis: further action based on LDL-cholesterol level

in which the screening took place: 3.8% had less than high school education, 31.8% had attended or graduated from college, 6.8% held master's degrees, and 57.6% had doctoral degrees.

With regard to lifestyle, 93% do not smoke and 40% are former smokers. Fifty-nine percent said they sometimes feel anxious, 29% often feel anxious, and 13% rarely feel anxious. In response to the question regarding vigorous conditioning exercise, 20.8% answered no, 41.6% exercise less than 3 times a week, and 37.6% exercise 3 times a week.

Fifty-four percent reported no health problems such as coronary artery disease, high blood pressure, diabetes, high cholesterol level or taking of estrogen in any form; this reflects primarily the young adult (19–35) group. Nearly 8% had one health problem and 1.5% reported two. There were missing data on 36% of the participants.

The questions regarding family history presented a different picture. Only 15.5% had no family history of heart attack or stroke before age 50, high blood pressure, diabetes, high cholesterol level, or coronary artery disease. Nineteen percent had one risk factor, 16.3% had two, 11.3% had three, and 12.2% had four or more. Again, a large number of the young adults did not know the family history. Slightly over one-third of this group (34.5%) had a family history of high cholesterol.

Body mass index (BMI) (Wt. (Kg.) + Ht (M^2), was calculated for the entire group; 26.6% of the females (19–35) and 28.8% of the males (19–35) had a high BMI. For the group age 36 and over 14.3% of the females and 9.7% of the males had a high BMI. This reflects a group who would be considered obese.

The responses to the questions about consumption of foods high in cholesterol indicated that only 25% of the group eat such foods more than one or two times per week. Twenty-four percent rarely or never eat foods high in cholesterol.

Classification of Participants

Cholesterol levels of the 888 participants with complete data were categorized according to the criteria approved by the expert panel and are shown in Table 2.

DISCUSSION

Nearly 30 percent (29.7%) of the total population screened could be categorized as having borderline high or high blood cholesterol levels. This percentage is greater than the 25% predicted by the cut-off values set by the NIH Consensus Conference. In the young white adult group, 12.8% fell into the borderline or high blood cholesterol category, again greater than the 10% expected. One explanation may be that those who participated in the screening did so because they thought they were in a high-risk category and wanted to check their cholesterol levels.

The effect of weight and marital status on mean cholesterol level (MCL) was significant in the 19–35 age group and the combined groups. The effect of educational level and smoking history on MCL was significant only when the combined groups were analyzed together. The amount of exercise and daily activity was inversely related to MCL in the 19–35 age group and the combined groups. The number of personal risk factors was related to MCL in the 36-and-over age group and in the combined groups, but not in the 19–35 age group. BMI was significantly related to MCL in all three groups.

Three of the variables which we thought would be related to MCL but were not significant in this population were anxiety, family health history, and diet scores.

The 61 participants with cholesterol levels ≥240 mg/dl were all contacted by telephone four months after the screening. Twenty-two (36%) of the participants had contacted their physicians for follow-up. Seven of these reported that they were put on medication to lower cholesterol level. Our follow-up found that many physicians were not aware of the revised criteria for classifying cholesterol and consequently responded inappropriately. Ten clients were told that their cholesterol levels were satisfactory and physicians

Table 2
Distribution of Cholesterol Levels

Age	Total Screened	Desirable BC Blood Cholesterol 200 mg/dl (%)	Borderline High Blood Cholesterol 200–239 mg/dl (%)	High Blood Cholesterol 240 mg/dl and up (%)
19–35	399	343 (82.7%)	40 (10.2%)	8 (2%)
36 and over	489	272 (56.2%)	159 (32.9%)	53 (11%)
TOTALS	888 (875)	615 (70.3%)	199 (22.7%)	61 (7%)
	(13 missing cases)			

didn't know why "those people were getting everyone so excited." The remaining five clients had not received any follow-up; they were encouraged to come to the NCFH for a recheck Two of the five have been reevaluated and both still had levels >240 mg/dl. They have been referred to a local laboratory for lipoprotein analysis.

We have had contact with many participants who were grouped in the borderline high blood cholesterol level (200–239 mg/dl); they have contacted the NCFH for diet information and rechecking of cholesterol. Several wanted to get their lipoprotein analysis even though their total cholesterol was <240 mg/dl.

LIMITATIONS

One important question regarding the value of mass cholesterol screening programs is whether they detect true elevations in serum cholesterol. Two factors may interfere with obtaining a true reading: the reliability of the portable machines in use, and known variation in cholesterol in individuals.

Although the availability of portable, easy-to-operate blood analyzers has the potential to make cholesterol screening available to more people, there have been questions raised about the reliability of such instruments (DeLong, DeLong, Wood, Lippel, & Rifkind, 1986). The Laboratory Standardization Panel of the National Cholesterol Education Program has recommended that accuracy of cholesterol measurement should not vary ±5% from the true value and, in terms of precision, the coefficients of variation (CV) should be 5% or less. They recommend that the instruments be standardized to either the CDC reference method or the National Reference System for cholesterol.

The BMD Reflotron® does meet all these criteria; it is standardized to the CDC reference method, the CV range is 2.3–3.8%, and the reported accuracy is within the ±5% range. We were able to get confirming readings from a clinical laboratory for those participants who went for lipoprotein analysis and in each case our screening measurement was within ±10 mg/dl of the measurement the laboratory obtained. We were aware of 16 such instances.

Recent studies have documented a seasonal variation in cholesterol measurement with higher readings being reported in winter and lower readings in spring (Gordon et al., 1987). Since this screening was done in early November there may be significantly higher levels than if we had screened in April. This seasonal shift could lead to a 30% increase in the number of referrals in winter versus spring.

The 1988 Expert Panel of the National Cholesterol Education Program reports that the total cholesterol level may fluctuate for an individual from day to day by one standard deviation which has been reported as 18 mg/dl.

Therefore, it is important to get more than one cholesterol measurement to assess accurately the serum cholesterol status in those individuals with borderline high and high cholesterol levels. We did recommend a recheck after one to four weeks for all those with cholesterol levels >220 mg/dl, but on follow-up contacts we found very few had complied with the recommendation.

Another limitation in this study is the fact that the participants do not represent a random sample. Those who participated were self-selected and were willing to pay a small fee to learn their cholesterol level, so they may be a more highly motivated group.

IMPLICATION FOR NURSING

From this experience it appears that there are a significant number of students, faculty, and staff in the 19–35 age range who have cholesterol levels >200 mg/dl and who could benefit from a program aimed at dietary modification and risk reduction. Both are areas in which nursing can intervene. The new recommendations for follow-up as established by the 1987 Expert Panel on Detection, Evaluation and Treatment of High Blood Cholesterol in Adults can serve as protocols for such nursing interventions.

It is also evident from our follow-up contacts that many physicians are not responding appropriately to the new guidelines and their patients are at risk. These people are concerned but don't know where to go for consultation. They might be interested in a program on campus which would be easily accessible. This group may need to be encouraged to take more responsibility for their own health. One barrier to their participation in a program in the NCFH is the medical insurance package at the university. Many of the young faculty and staff belong to a local HMO and the HMO will not pay for testing or counseling done outside the organization.

In summary, it is clear that there is a role for nursing in the detection, evaluation, and nonpharmaceutical treatment of high blood cholesterol in adults.

REFERENCES

DeLong, D.M., DeLong, E.R., Wood, P.D., Lippel, K., & Rifkind, B.M. (1986). A comparison of methods for the estimation of plasma low- and very low-density lipoprotein cholesterol. The Lipid Research Clinics Prevalence Study. *Journal of the American Medical Association, 256,* 2372–2377.

Gordon, D.J., Trost, D.C., Hyde, J., Whaley, F.S., Hannan, P.J., Jacob, D.R., & Ekelund, L. (1987). Seasonal cholesterol cycles: The Lipid Research Clinics Coronary Primary Prevention Trial placebo group. *Circulation, 76,* 1224–1231.

Lipid Research Clinics Program. (1984a). The Lipid Research Clinics Coronary Primary Prevention Trial results: I. Reduction in the incidence of coronary heart disease. *Journal of the American Medical Association, 251,* 351–364.

Lipid Research Clinics Program. (1984b). The Lipid Research Clinics Coronary Primary Prevention Trial results: II. The relationship of reduction in incidence of coronary heart disease to cholesterol lowering. *Journal of the American Medical Association, 251,* 365–374.

Martin, M.J., Hulley, S.B., Browner, W.S., Kuller, L.H., & Wentworth, D. (1986). Serum cholesterol, blood pressure, and mortality: Implications from a cohort of 361, 662 men. *Lancet, 2,* 933–936.

Report from the Laboratory Standardization Panel of the National Cholesterol Education Program. (1988). Current status of blood cholesterol measurement in clinical laboratories in the United States. *Clinical Chemistry, 34,* 193–201.

Report of the Expert Panel of the National Cholesterol Education Program (1988). *Detection, evaluation, and treatment of high blood cholesterol in adults.* Washington, DC: Public Health Service.

Stamler, Wentworth, D., & Neaton, J.D. for the Multiple Risk Factor Intervention Trial Research Group. (1986). Is relationship between serum cholesterol and risk of premature death from coronary heart disease continuous and graded? *Journal of the American Medical Association, 256,* 2823–2828.

BIBLIOGRAPHY

American Heart Association. (1986). Dietary guidelines for healthy American adults: A statement for physicians and health professionals by the Nutrition Committee, American Heart Association. *Circulation, 74*(6), 1465A–1468A.

Bausell, R.B., & Pruitt, R.H. (1986). Cholesterol knowledge, avoidance, and monitoring among the American public. *Heart and Lung, 15,* 543–547.

Becker, D.M., & Wilder, L.B. (1987). Nutritional and pharmacological approaches to hypercholesterolemia.*Cardio-Vascular Nursing, 25*(3)12–16.

DeLong, D.M., DeLong, E.R., Wood, P.D., Lippel, K., & Rifkind, B.M. (1986).

A comparison of methods for the estimation of plasma low- and very low-density lipoprotein cholesterol. The Lipid Research Clinics Prevalence Study. *Journal of the American Medical Association, 256,* 2372–2377.

Gordon, D.J., Trost, D.C., Hyde, J., Whaley, F.S., Hannan, P.J., Jacob, D.R., & Ekelund, L. (1987). Seasonal cholesterol cycles: The Lipid Research Clinics Coronary Primary Prevention Trial placebo group. *Circulation, 76,* 1224–1231.

Gotto, A.M. Jr, Bierman, E.L., Conner, W.E., Ford, C.H., Frantz, I.D. Jr., Glueck, C.J., Grundy, S.M., & Little, J.A. (1984). Recommendations for treatment of hyperlipidemia in adults. A joint statement of the Nutrition Committee and the Council on Arteriosclerosis. *Circulation, 69,* 1067A–1090A.

Greenland, P., Levenkron, J.C., Radley, M.G., Baggs, J.G., Manchester, R.A., & Bowley, N.L. (1987). Feasibility of large-scale cholesterol screening: Experience with a portable capillary-blood testing device. *American Journal of Public Health, 77,* 73–75.

Grundy, S.M. (1986). Cholesterol and coronary heart disease, a new era. *Journal of the American Medical Association, 256,* 2849–2858.

Keys, A., Anderson, J.T., & Grande, F. (1965). Serum cholesterol response to changes in the diet. *Metabolism, 14,* 747–787.

Koch, T.R., Mehta, U., Lee, H., Aziz, J., Temel, S., Donion, J., & Sherwin, R. (1987). Bias and precision of cholesterol analysis by physician's office analyzers. *Clinical Chemistry, 33*(12), 2262–2267.

Lipid Research Clinics Program (1984a). The Lipid Research Clinics Coronary Primary Prevention Trial results: I. Reduction in the incidence of coronary heart disease. *Journal of the American Medical Association, 251,* 351–364.

Lipid Research Clinics Program (1984b). The Lipid Research Clinics Coronary Primary Prevention Trial results: II. The relationship of reduction in incidence of coronary heart disease to cholesterol lowering. *Journal of the American Medical Association, 251,* 365–374.

Martin, M.J., Hulley, S.B., Browner, W.S., Kuller, L.H., & Wentworth, D. (1986). Serum cholesterol, blood pressure, and mortality: Implications from a cohort of men 361, 662 men. *Lancet, 2,* 933–936.

National Institutes of Health Statement. (1985). Lowering blood cholesterol to prevent heart disease. *Journal of the American Medical Association, 253,* 2080–2086.

Reed, T., Wagoner, D.K., Donahue, R.P., & Kuller, L.H. (1986). Young adult cholesterol as a predictor of familial ischemic heart disease. *Preventive Medicine, 15,* 292–303.

Report from the Laboratory Standardization Panel of the National Cholesterol Education Program (1988). Current status of blood cholesterol measurement in clinical laboratories in the United States. *Clinical Chemistry, 34,* 193–201.

Report of the Expert Panel of the National Cholesterol Education Program (1988). *Detection, evaluation, and treatment of high blood cholesterol in adults.* Washington, DC: Public Health Service.

Roberts, L. (1987). Measuring cholesterol is as tricky as lowering it. *Science, 258,* 482–483.

Stamler, Wentworth, D., & Neaton, J.D. for the Multiple Risk Factor Intervention Trial Research Group (1986). Is relationship between serum cholesterol and risk of premature death from coronary heart disease continuous and graded? *Journal of the American Medical Association, 256,* 2823–2828.

Suter, P.M., Superko, R., Wood, P., & Suter, N. (1987). Fingerstick technique preferred in blood sampling for cholesterol. *American Journal for Public Health, 102,* 453.

Wynder, E.L., Field, F., & Haley, N. (1986). Population screening for cholesterol determination. *Journal of the American Medical Association, 256,* 2839–2842.

8

Models of Academic Nurse-Managed Centers

Zana Rae Higgs, EdD, RN

Since the late 1970s, faculty members at the Intercollegiate Center for Nursing Education (ICNE) in Spokane, Washington have developed clinical learning opportunities for undergraduate nursing students outside of the auspices of existing health care agencies (Mealey, 1981; Higgs, 1985). Through these experiences, a number of issues have arisen including continuity of care, coordination time required on the part of faculty involved, and funding to support services provided. It was determined that an understanding of the experiences faculty of other schools of nursing have had with the development of such learning experiences was needed prior to formalizing these clinical arrangements into an ongoing health care system.

Such faculty-created and -organized clinical learning experiences have been termed "academic nurse-managed centers" (NMC) or "nursing clinics". An extensive review of the literature provided descriptions of individual NMCs and some discussions of perspectives of faculty involved in this movement. Three research endeavors were found (Barger, 1986a–d; Boettcher, 1985; Fehring, Schulte, & Riesch, 1986). The problem facing the ICNE was to develop a clearer understanding of this phenomenon. Thus, this investigator performed a study to determine issues related to the development and maintenance of NMCs and develop models of NMCs based on this descriptive data.

Findings regarding characteristics of NMCs and issues to be addressed by faculty and nursing education administrators developing an NMC have been reported elsewhere (Higgs, 1988). The purpose of this article is to describe models of NMCs that arose from analysis of their defining characteristics.

METHOD

The study entailed a descriptive survey research approach using telephone interviews. Schools with NMCs were identified from the review of literature and registration lists from workshops on NMCs. Faculty participating in the NMC movement provided additional names during telephone interviews. Eighty-seven schools of nursing were contacted and interviews were conducted with faculty from 65 schools with NMCs and 12 schools planning or interested in developing such centers.

A semi-structured interview schedule was developed to determine characteristics of existing NMCs and the issues faced by faculty working with these centers. Selection of topics for discussion during the interview was based on the literature review. Additional questions were added to the survey as phone interviews progressed and issues began to surface. Content analysis was performed on data acquired through telephone interviews.

FINDINGS

The variation found among academic nurse-managed centers demonstrates the creativity of faculty as they have sought to address issues of needed student learning experiences, faculty practice opportunities, and commitment to serve underserved populations across the United States. NMCs may replace university health services or provide additional services to the university and surrounding community within space provided on the university campus. They may be housed in mobile vans, churches, missions, senior centers, senior housing complexes, daycare centers, and elsewhere. NMCs are evolving, developing, and expanding. However, those that were developed under a major grant beyond the financial means of the university and community have reduced the services offered and the hours of operation.

Because of this wide variation, it was difficult to formulate distinct models without overlapping boundaries. However, there were certain characteristics that, when taken together, allowed NMCs to be categorized into four models. Given the lack of precision of content analysis, each NMC in a category may not meet exactly all the criteria of each defining characteristic of that model. However, this investigator would suggest the emergence of four relatively distinct models. The defining characteristics of these models include (1) number of hours open per week, (2) personnel, (3) primary scope of nursing practice, (4) degree of emphasis on instruction versus service, (5) amount of noncompensated care provided, (6) student involvement, (7) coordination, (8) funding, (9) continuity, (10) faculty practice, and (11) competition in health care market. The number of sites, type of site, specific client population served, and specific services rendered were characteristics that did not prove to be relevant in categorizing NMCs. Table 1 outlines the four models. In the following discussion, each of the four models of NMCs is described and the proportion of the sample which fit that model is noted.

Table 1
Models of Academic Nurse-managed Centers

Characteristics	Model I	Model II	Model III	Model IV
Hours/week	Less Than 40	Less Than 40	40	40
Personnel	Volunteer	Volunteer + Paid	Faculty Paid	Paid
Practice Focus	Generalist	Generalist	Advance	Advance
Education vs. Service	Education	Education	Both	Service +
Noncompensated	All	Most	Limited	None
Students	Undergraduate	Undergraduate +	Graduate +	Graduate
Coordinator	None	Limited	Yes	Yes
Continuity	An Issue	An Issue	Yes	Yes
Funding	In-Kind	Generate Some	Fee +	Fee +
Faculty Practice	No, No Reward	Some, No Reward	Yes + Reward	Yes + Reward
Competition	None	None	Yes	Yes

Model I: 34% (22 Programs)

Model I NMCs are open less than 40 hours per week. Personnel includes only faculty during instructional time or is heavily dependent upon faculty, student, and possibly community nurse volunteers. It has no paid staff and faculty are usually not nurse-practitioners. The primary focus of the NMC is generalist-level primary care. Its purpose is instructional, resulting in a community service. Its clients are the underserved who receive noncompensated care. Competition for market share is not an issue. Student involvement is primarily at the undergraduate level, especially for health assessment, community health nursing, and well-child care learning experiences. If graduate students are involved, they are not from practitioner or clinician programs, rather they are assigned to do their student teaching as nursing education majors or perform some nursing service administration project. There is no assigned coordinator. The faculty members involved in the NMC for clinical instruction provide the coordination as an overload and faculty workload adjustments are rarely made to account for additional time this requires. Lack of assigned coordinator time leads to difficulty maintaining the center, difficulty generating additional financial and community support, and burnout on the part of faculty involved. Funding is from institutional budgets for faculty instructional positions. Little revenue is generated by the NMC. In-kind support from the university and/or community agencies sustains the program. There are limited or no contracts for services. Therefore, ongoing funding is a considerable concern of those involved and mechanisms are being considered to acquire additional funding. Continuity is an issue unless the school has summer courses. Ongoing services are not provided during summers and breaks. However, faculty may volunteer time to keep the clinic open during limited hours of service. Practice as a component of the faculty role is not rewarded in the university promotion and tenure policies nor is it an expected activity of nursing faculty.

Model II: 15% (10 Programs)

These NMCs are open less than 40 hours per week. Personnel is comprised of instructional faculty that often includes nurse practitioners. The center may have either a part-time RN/clerk paid by a community agency or faculty release time for coordination. The center may also use faculty volunteers. Faculty who are practitioners are beginning to use these NMCs for some of their practice time. The primary focus is generalist-level primary care with the limited addition of advanced scopes of practice. These NMCs continue to exist primarily for instructional purposes, but there is an increased focus on service.

There is some change in client populations. In addition to noncompensated care, there is a broadening of the population base particularly in states where nurses with advanced practice credentials have prescriptive authority and direct reimbursement through their own individual provider number. Therefore, some services may be covered by Medicare, Medicaid, and other third-party payers. Also, the NMC is more likely to contract with organizations to provide services for a fee. Clients are more likely to be asked to donate or be charged a minimal fee for services. Funding arrangement remains an issue. Most of the financial help still comes through in-kind university and community support. However, these centers are beginning to generate a small portion of the funds needed to sustain the program themselves. Undergraduate students remain the bulk of students deriving learning experiences through these NMCs. There may also be nurse practitioner graduate students. These centers are more likely to have some portion of a faculty member's time set aside for coordination of the center; that is, a specific amount of faculty time for coordination activities is incorporated into the faculty workload with a commensurate reduction in instructional responsibilities. This faculty member then serves as the preceptor for undergraduate/graduate students. Because of the advanced scope of practice, faculty may have medical protocol backup. However, they are not usually seen as competing with physicians for a market share of patient care. Continuity remains an issue with faculty who volunteer time or use practice time for coverage. These NMCs are more likely to have part-time paid staff coverage during summers. Faculty practice is valued and encouraged but not rewarded in tenure and promotion decisions.

Model III 34% (22 Programs)

These NMCs are open 40 hours per week, or faculty members have their own private practice to which students are assigned for learning experiences. These centers are well established and have a stable base of operation. Personnel for these NMCs usually consists of nurse practitioner faculty with greater balance between instructional time and private practice time. These faculty members serve as preceptors for a small number of nurse practitioner graduate students. As an alternative, these NMCs have generalist faculty who have developed a well-established, ongoing program of services, or there is a combination of these two approaches. The emphasis tends to be on advanced practice which requires meeting additional licensure/certification requirements for the level of nursing care provided. In some cases, services (i.e., service for a fee, and not volunteer community service) tends to overshadow the instructional focus of the NMC. A larger percentage of clients have compensable care, especially through Medicare and Medicaid. These services require medical backup and protocols as would be expected of a nurse practitioner's private practice or a university medical center clinic.

These NMCs may be seen as being in competition with physicians, and market share may be an issue. On the other hand, if the services rendered continue within the generalist scope of nursing practice there may be no competition with the medical community. However, even performing sports physicals for school children may be considered by pediatricians as a competitive move. Most of these NMCs shift their educational focus to graduate students. For those that do not, the well-established, extensive program offers experiences for multiple levels of undergraduate students and courses. There is a coordinator, either a paid position or one half-time joint faculty appointment. The NMCs usually have secretarial or clerical help, especially related to billing activities. In addition to in-kind and instructional budget support, there is some type of payment system for services. There is also some noncompensated care provided, and payment for services is insufficient to make the NMC totally self-sustaining. Therefore, overhead and in some cases a portion of personnel costs must be maintained by the university, community agencies, or grant funds.

Continuity is not usually a problem as the nurse practitioners maintain an ongoing practice or the NMC provides year-round services. Faculty practice is valued, often required, and is more likely to be rewarded in tenure and promotion considerations. As an alternative, a clinical track has been established.

Model IV: 17% (11 Programs)

These NMCs are established as nonprofit or for-profit businesses. They are open 40 hours per week, and may be independent private faculty practices. Faculty have advanced licensure or certification, for example, as nurse practitioners, or are selling primary-care services, particularly health education and consultation services. The focus has shifted to advanced practice, or if it remains at a generalist level, the NMC is typically a private-duty or home health care business. In addition, the focus is on service for compensation, rather than instruction. When students are involved, there are only a limited number of nurse practitioner graduate students, or undergraduate students are assigned to provide reimbursable services as in any health facility in which students are placed for clinical experiences. Frequently, these NMCs are located in the clinic facility of a university medical center. Client services are charged to Medicare, Medicaid, or third-party payers. In instances of consultation and health education, fees are charged for services rendered. Whatever the arrangement, a payment system has been established for all services. With in-kind support, particularly for space and overhead, these NMCs are breaking even, self-supporting, or income-generating. There is some concern over the potential expectations for these NMCs to generate income back into the university as do medical faculty in university hospitals. Some type of coordination is required to develop marketable services and bill clients. Continuity is not a concern as these centers are ongoing businesses. Faculty practice is valued, often required, and rewarded in promotion and tenure criteria. As an alternative, a "clinical practice track" has been created for faculty interested in focusing on instruction and direct clinical practice in their faculty role.

SUMMARY

It is unclear as to what degree these models form developmental stages. It is clear that each model has its strengths and areas of concern. Community needs, faculty expertise and interests, educational focus of the school of nursing, and the university's mission and goals are major determinants in identifying which model is most appropriate for any given school of nursing. Much can be learned from the experiences of other schools, which will be helpful for those already involved in the NMC movement of those faculty and schools of nursing considering developing such a school of nursing-managed health care service.

REFERENCES

Barger, S. (1986a). Academic nurse-managed centers: Issues of implementation. *Family and Community Health, 9,* 12–22.

Barger, S. (1986b). Academic nursing centers: A demographic profile. *Journal of Professional Nursing, 2*(4), 246–251.

Barger, S. (1986c). Nursing center: From concept to reality. *Journal of Community Health Nursing, 3*(4), 175–182.

Barger, S. (1986d). Personnel issues of academic nurse-managed centers: The pitfalls and the potential. *Nurse Educator, 11*(3), 28–33.

Boettcher, J. (1985). *Nursing centers in academic and faculty job satisfaction,* (PhD Dissertation). Austin, TX: University of Texas, Austin.

Fehring, R., Schulte, J., & Riesch, S. (1986). Toward a definition of nurse-managed centers. *Journal of Community Health Nursing, 3*(2), 59-67.

Higgs, Z. (1985). Carry the water to the desert. *Journal of Professional Nursing, 1*(4), 217–220.

Higgs, Z. (1988). The academic nurse-managed center movement: A survey report. *Journal of Professional Nursing, 4*(6) 422–429.

Mealey, A. (1981). Provision of a multi-range program for clients in a downtown hotel by baccalaureate nursing students. *Journal of Advanced Nursing, 11*(3), 295–301.

9

Community Wellness Outreach: Family Health through Empowerment

Marjorie Buchanan, MS, RN
Patricia L. Gerrity, PhD, RN

Community Wellness Outreach (CWO) is a unique and effective collaboration between community leaders and the nursing profession in Philadelphia. CWO promotes family well-being through an empowerment model of health care. Philadelphia's broad range of socioeconomic groups, rich ethnic and cultural diversity, and excellent health resources, offer elements of strength as well as significant barriers to family health associated with each of these factors. The efforts fo CWO focus on empowering young families who have had difficulty addressing their health needs successfully, yet who possess the potential for change. Acknowledging and enhancing strengths, and identifying and reducing barriers to effective care enables families to formulate positive approaches to their health needs.

FAMILIES IN NEED

The Mayor's Commission on Infant Mortality (1985) reports that low income childbearing families in Philadelphia are at great risk with regard to their childrens' health. Many have not sought or have inconsistently utilized available resources for health promotion/disease prevention services. Recurring episodic illness, frequent injuries, evidence of growth and development delays in children, poor management of chronic health problems, and family neglect and abuse seen in ambulatory care settings and hospital emergency rooms support the Commission's findings.

Health knowledge and skill deficits, a crisis orientation toward health care, difficulties in accessing the system, and numerous challenging social factors underlie the problems encountered by health professionals. Moreover, examination from a transcultural perspective reveals that the health care system itself is a contributor to the health care difficulties of families. Complex scheduling procedures, a highly technological environment, and unfamiliar medical terminology, all heighten the challenges of the family as client.

Leininger (1984) defines culture as "the learned, shared, and transmitted values, beliefs, norms, and lifeway practices of a particular group that guides thinking, decisions, and actions in patterned ways" (p. 209). This term can be applied to consumers and providers alike in today's health care system. Each has their own way of doing things, their own language, and because of these differences, a communication gap develops between them and compromises health care (Figure 1). A communication gap blocks client access to the health care provider and vice versa. The culture and language of poverty, ethnic differences, and difficult life experiences contrast sharply with the language and culture of the professional and scientific health system, social service system, and often the larger community system as well. Cultural care

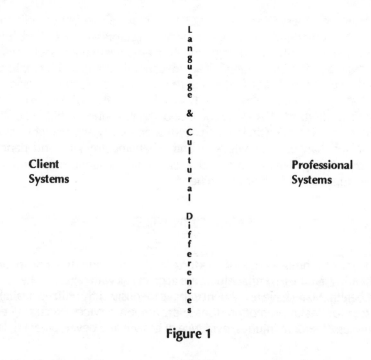

Figure 1

preservation where possible, accommodation as appropriate, and repatterning as necessary, are needed for clients and providers alike.

ORGANIZATION AND ADMINISTRATION

CWO is comprised of a board of directors, an executive director, an advisory panel, and program directors. The board of directors includes members of the original organizing group, and representatives of the target communities. The executive director assists, facilitates, and supports program initiatives by identifying potential resources that will generate funds. She also serves as a liaison between the program directors and the board. Members of the advisory panel serve as consultants to the board, the executive director, and the programs.

The two community health nursing faculty serve as the program directors by virtue of their established relationships with communities in need—specifically, two low-income black neighborhoods and the growing southeast Asian refugee population in Philadelphia. Whereas faculty are responsible for program development, registered nurses in the two RN-to-BSN programs implement the program objectives. This is consistent with the learning objectives established by the respective educational institutions. The students' learning is enhanced as their efforts move beyond academic exercises designed merely to meet course requirements. Rather, involvement in such initiatives engages them in community life to such an extent that they invest expertise, creativity, and energy well beyond course expectations. Learning outcomes reflect that students have moved beyond their acute-care orientation to broader definitions of both health care and the nursing role. This experience enables them to deliver care which is beyond the boundaries of traditional institutional settings.

EMPOWERMENT MODEL OF CARE

An empowerment model of care serves as the organizing framework for program efforts. Kantor (1977) describes power as the ability to get things done, to mobilize resources, and to get and use whatever is needed to achieve the goals that have been established. To be empowered is to have control over the conditions that make action possible, thus to be able to do and have what one needs and wants. This is consistent with the Ottawa Charter for Action to Achieve Health for All By the Year 2000 and Beyond (World Health Organization, et al., 1986), which states:

> Health promotion is the process of enabling people to increase control over, and to improve, their health. To reach a state of complete . . . well being, an individual or group must be able to identify and to realize aspirations, to satisfy needs, and to change or cope with the environment. Health is therefore, seen as a resource for everyday life, not the objective of living. Health is a positive concept emphasizing social and personal resources as well as physical capacities. Therefore, health promotion is not the responsibility of the health sector but goes beyond healthy lifestyles to well being.

The means by which well-being is enhanced are advocacy, enablement, and mediation for health promotion. These actions are designed to build healthy public policy, create supportive environments, strengthen community action, develop personal skills, and reorient health services (Figure 2). Success in application of the empowerment model of care was determined to lie in its *simultaneous* application to families, human service providers/organizations, and the larger community. Simultaneous application recognizes, acknowledges, and facilitates reduction of the cultural gap (Leininger, 1986) (Figure 3).

IMPACT

Initial evaluation of the CWO programs indicated that benefits w ere realized by clients and organizations for whom the programs were desigred. Families have begun to increase the effectiveness of their health strategie s. They have an increased awareness of the resources available to them, a etter understanding of the appropriate use of the different levels of care, and they no longer use services on an emergency-only basis.

The health care providers are becoming more sensitive to the cultural differences of their clients and have gained a heightened awareness of the overall needs of their target populations. Faculty from the two schools have found that the collaborative effort of community leaders and nursing professionals not only provides a source of encouragement for their efforts in the community, but also helps enhance and broaden their teaching abilities. The faculty have brought the students from the two programs together at least one time each semester to share their clinical experiences. In addition, students have independently consulted each other when their projects have over-

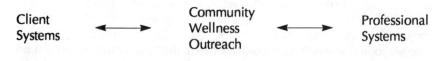

Figure 2

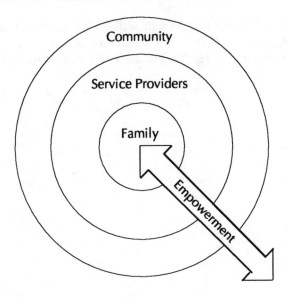

Figure 3

lapped or addressed similar populations. One of the most exciting outcomes has been the increased awareness and appreciation for the present and potential role of nursing in addressing the health needs of the community. Health care providers from local agencies, neighborhood representatives, and nurses from CWO have begun to meet together to address local problems. As a result, plans are now underway to establish a nursing center that is a collaborative venture between the two universities.It will then be possible to expand program development to address the needs of populations beyond those presently being served.

REFERENCES

Kantor, R.M. (1977). *Men and women of the corporation.* New York: Basic Books.

Leininger, M. (1984). Transcultural care—diversity and universality: A theory of nursing. *Nursing and Health Care.* April, 209–212.

The Mayor's Commission on Infant Mortality. (1985). *Recommendations for the reduction of infant mortality in Philadelphia.* November, Philadelphia, PA.

World Health Organization, Health and Welfare Canada, Canadian Public Health Association. (1986). *Ottawa charter for health promotion.* International Conference on Health Promotion. Ottawa, Canada, November 21, 1986.

10

A Nursing Model of Health Care:
A 10-Year Trend Analysis

Ellamae Branstetter, PhD, RN
Elizabeth Holman, MS, RN

Since 1977, the Community Health Services Nursing Practice Center of the College of Nursing at Arizona State University has been offering health care to the citizens of Scottsdale, Tempe, and the general Phoenix metropolitan area. Generally referred to as "the clinic," the center originally was developed by nursing faculty and students through a USPHS Division of Nursing Advanced Nurse Training grant award, but for the past six years has been maintained by the college through fee collections, university support, cooperative arrangements with the City of Scottsdale and the Maricopa County Health Department, and through contributions from various charitable groups in the community.

In this discussion we will briefly review the history of the clinic and present a 10-year analysis of trends in selected operational variables, utilization of services, client characteristics, and faculty/student participation.

The clinic was established primarily to develop (in collaboration with the community) affordable nursing health care services for a community that needed and wanted those services, while at the same time serving as a clinical and educational practice site for faculty and students. A further purpose was to involve faculty, students, and segments of the larger community in the development and continuation of those health services. This approach to providing health care features the nurse as the primary provider, and thus was called a "nursing model of health care." As we defined the model in 1977, the nurse assumes the primary responsibility in the planning, provision, and evaluation of health care services.

This model focuses on the prevention of health problems, promotion of health, and health maintenance activities. The model also includes treatment of minor illnesses and appropriate referrals for persons with complex health problems that require medical care. The nurse functions both independently and collaboratively, and is a planner and initiator of care as well as coordinator of continuing care. One of the reasons for the college of nursing's sponsorship is that of providing educational experiences for students, and this approach provides an opportunity for actual demonstration of innovative nursing roles with an opportunity for the student to become an active partner in the expression of these roles.

The physician's role in this model, as it was set into operation in 1977, was that of consultant, advisor, instructor, prescription writer, protocol reviewer, and only occasionally, provider of health services. Since our purpose was to emphasize what the *nurse* could do, the physician's role in providing services to clients was minimized. Later, we needed to increase fee collections, we examined productivity of all staff, and physicians as well as nurse providers were hence expected to provide services to clients. That pattern continues today, with physicians dealing mainly with those clients with more complex health problems.

Since 1977, the nursing model of health care has been the unique characteristic of the clinic's services in our community, for in other health services (both private and public) the medical model of health care prevails. Clinic services were initiated during the summer of 1977. Within a three-month period, full-time services were in effect from 8 a.m. to 5 p.m. Monday through Friday. That schedule remains in effect today, with the addition of selected evening sessions. It is important to mention that before services were initiated in May 1977, both a formal and an informal survey of community health needs were conducted. Informally, faculty met with local citizens' groups, City of Scottsdale personnel, and other human services professionals to determine their perceptions of specific immediate needs. These meetings, along with data from the community survey revealed outstanding needs in:

- treatment of minor illnesses (especially for children)
- family planning
- well-child clinics
- immunization programs

These programs were introduced first, with a general health-promotion, family health orientation throughout. A statement of philosophy was developed early in the project, and remains today as a guiding force in deliberations concerning the direction of the clinic.

Figures 1–14 graphically portray selected trends during the period 1977–1987. Although the clinic was actually begun in 1974 on a part-time, volunteer basis, the computer information system was not developed until 1978, so the reconstruction of events, client information, and encounters was not easily retrievable for the period beginning in 1974. Those early years were very important in preparing the community for the introduction of full-time nursing services, mainly due to the efforts of one person, Marjorie Hauenstein, the nurse-coordinator during those years. Her rapport with the community paved the way for the programs introduced in 1977.

PROGRAM OFFERINGS

In addition to preventive services, health promotion activities and health maintenance, we have offered health restoration services, or treatment of

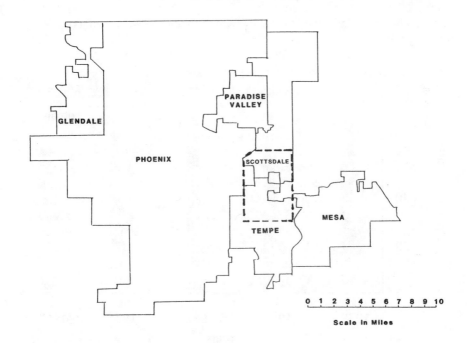

Figure 1
Area Served in 1987

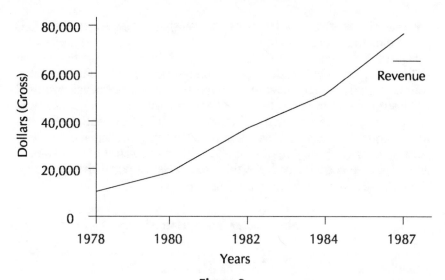

Figure 2
Revenues: Client Collections

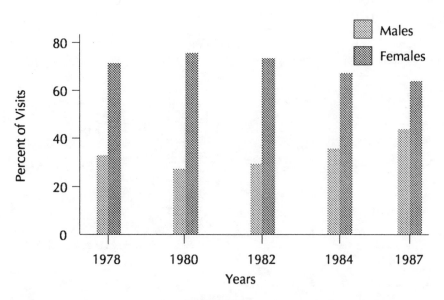

Figure 3
Percent of Clinic Visits by Gender of Client

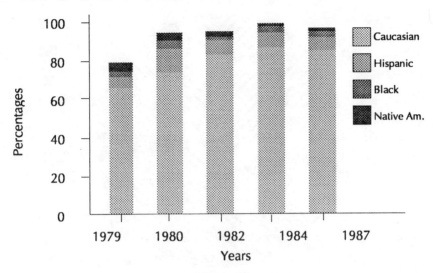

Figure 4
Ethnicity of Clients 1979–1987

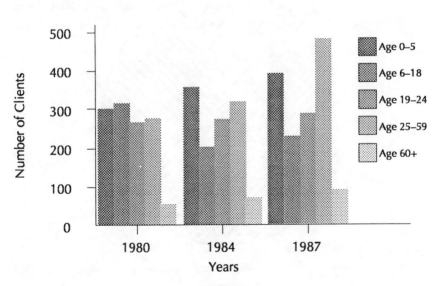

Figure 5
Age of Clients Recruited 1980/84/87

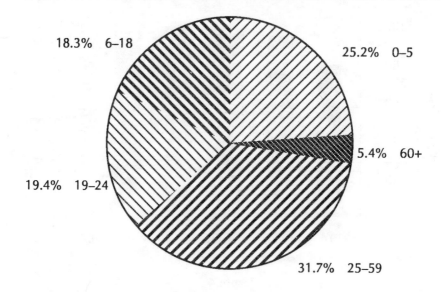

Figure 6
Age of Client Profile Summary 1980/84/87

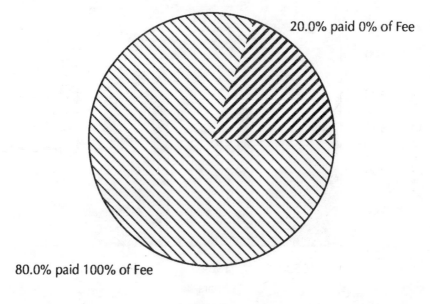

Figure 7
Clinic Service Fees: Percentage Paid by Clients 1987

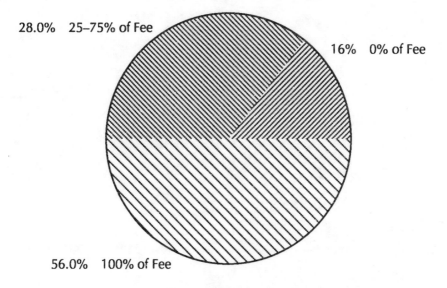

Figure 8
Clinic Service Fees: Percentage Paid by Clients 1984

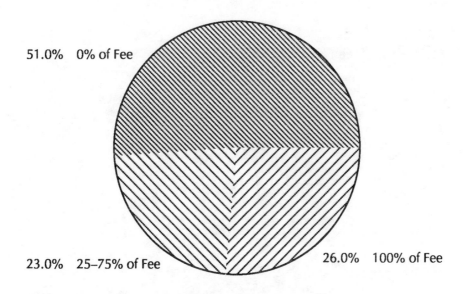

Figure 9
Clinic Service Fees: Percentage Paid by Clients 1982

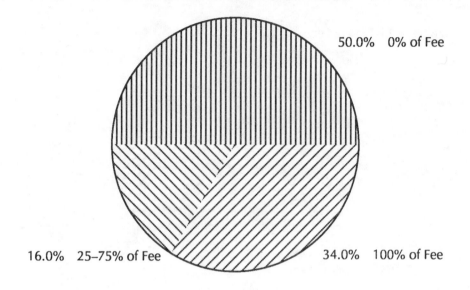

Figure 10
Clinic Service Fees: Percentage Paid by Clients 1980

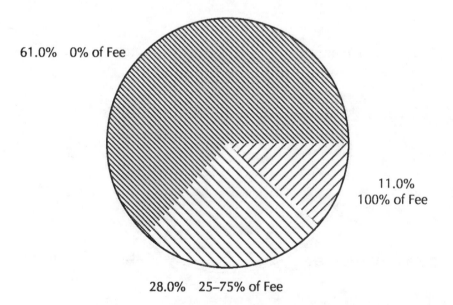

Figure 11
Clinic Service Fees: Percentage Paid by Clients 1978

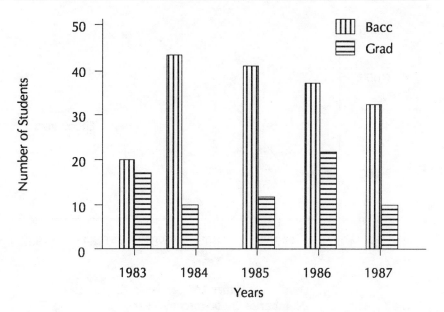

Figure 12
Nursing Students' Participation 1983–87

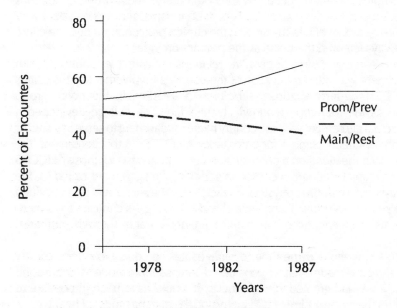

Figure 13
Percent of Encounters by Focus of Visit 1978/82/87

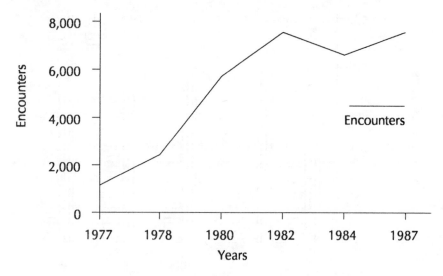

Figure 14
Number of Encounters by Year

noncomplex illnesses, needed by the community. These program offerings are congruent with the educational needs of students, and are consistent with the nursing model of health care and the clinic's philosophy. Thus, the clinic has always featured the nurse as the primary provider.

Two years ago, our cooperative relationship with the County Health Department was altered because of the county's involvement in the state's AHCCCS program (Arizona's substitute for Medicaid), the notch group known as the Maricopa (county) Health Plan. The college developed a contractual agreement with the county health department to serve as a site for the care of clients eligible for care under AHCCCS; in this agreement, the county paid the clinic on a per-visit (and per-capita) basis for those AHCCCS and Maricopa Health Plan clients. In addition, the agreement called for the placement of a half-time physician in the clinic. The agreement thus provided payment for some clients who were already utilizing the clinic on a reduced-fee basis, and enhanced the clinic's financial status through increased revenue.

In 1988, when it came time to renegotiate the county contract, county health officials made what we considered unreasonable requests for time and space. If we had granted these requests, it would have been impossible to maintain the existing clinic philosophy and the nursing model of health care. Instead, the medical model would have prevailed. After many unsuccessful attempts to negotiate with city and county officials, it was decided that the best chance for survival was to relocate to a shopping center about four blocks from the original site. The new location was accessible and convenient for continuing clients and provided optimum potential for recruiting new clients. Additionally, the owner of the building agreed to make necessary renovations, and university officials gave approval and temporary financial assistance. Clients were notified of the move to the new quarters, and in October 1988, services were continued at the new location with only minimal disruption.

Now, one year later, we are pleased that the move was necessary. Services and income have increased, and the clinic is well on its way to being self-supporting within the next year or so. This success can be attributed to an active marketing program; quality services which are needed by the community; an accessible and highly visible location; a supportive community; excellent management; an efficient staff; and helpful support from faculty, students, and university administration.

11

Geriatric Education and Health Management Clinic: Synergy in a Nursing Center

Sara Jane H. Anderson, MSN, ANP, RN

HISTORY

The Geriatric Education and Health Management Center (GEHMC) began as a voluntary effort in January 1987 as a cooperative effort of the University of New Mexico College of Nursing and the Albuquerque Office of Senior Affairs (AOSA). The AOSA provides space, telephones, and a yearly budget for desk supplies. A three-year training grant from the U.S. Department of Health and Human Services, Division of Nursing was received in November 1988. The grant funds student nursing-home experience, geriatric curriculum development, and continuing education. Funding from the grant also provides for a project director, adult nurse practitioner, gero-psychiatric nursing specialist, equipment, and consultation.

FUNCTION

The goal of the GEHMC is to increase health-promoting self-care among our 150 enrolled clients and the Highland Senior Center population. Our center is located in an ethnically and socioeconomically diverse east downtown area one mile from the university on old U.S. Route 66. We have use of a 20-by 30-foot room divided into cubicles by portable screens. The room houses our 3 filing cabinets, an examination table, and a large shelf. We have a desk and small table with 2 typewriters in the front lobby and reception area. From noon to 4 p.m. every Friday our main room is usually filled with 5 faculty members, 8 students, and 12 or more clients who are reporting for appointments; or requesting earlier appointments, information, immediate assessment of a recent change in vision, or to have a back rub. The nurses are evaluating an urgent concern, doing a finger-stick glucose, or shuffling appointments, trying to meet all demands, Meanwhile, the screen around the table where the back rub is being given is threatening to fall over, and 4 people from the AOSA swimming program have shown up unexpectedly for swimming program physicals! A first-time visitor to the center or a consumer advisory board member stopping by to see how things are doing might well wonder: "How does it work? Why do people keep coming to this wild place? Why are they willing to subject themselves to this chaos?" In what follows I will suggest one plausible reason for our center's success: synergy in the nurse, client, and environment subsystems of the GEHM system.

SYNERGY

Synergy is the combined or cooperative action or force. In our case, the goal of this action is the ordering of various events and processes to promote ongoing system function. The elements contributing to synergy in each subsystem are: energy (power), enjoyment (positive affect), and enthusiasm (motivation) (Figure 1).

NURSE

How are each of the elements of synergy reflec.ed in the nurse subsystem? First, energy is manifested in the backgrounds of the three project staff members. This includes community health, gero-psychiatric, and adult-practitioner nursing experience. During the last nine years, staff members have also started two other nursing clinics and submitted seven proposals to state and national agencies which were not funded. It is something we have all wanted to do for a long time!

Other nurse-subsystem energy sources include knowledge and skill in the nursing process (Carpenito, 1987) and Orem self-care nursing conceptualizations (Orem, 1985). The relationship between therapeutic communication, self-concept enhancement, goal contracting, and self-care is the intervention

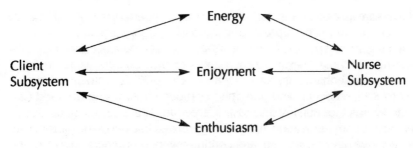

Figure 1
Synergy in Client–Nurse System in Senior Center Environment

and research thrust. Clarifying concepts of care, self, and nursing, and communicating them effectively to students, colleagues, and the public constitute professional life goals of the author.

Data collection tools include: Multiassessment Inventory (Lawton, 1982), Mood Assessment Scale (Yesavage, 1983), Mini Mental State (Folstein, 1975), Rosenberg Self Esteem Scale (Mangen, 1982), Health Risk Appraisal (Carter Center, 1988), and a self-care behaviors inventory in process by GEHM staff. Diagnosing follows the latest guidelines of the North American Nursing Diagnosis Association. Students have a two-credit course dealing exclusively with nursing process in their first clinical semester, so they are well oriented to this approach.

In the planning phase we use a goal contracting form, the Personal Wellness Plan and the Goal Attainment Scaling Technique (Schultz, 1979). This form is based on the attainment of levels in relation to each nursing diagnosis. Level one is the most unfavorable treatment outcome likely, and level five is the best anticipated success with treatment. The other three levels are spaced evenly between these extremes. An example of a scale for hours-per-week at a senior center for a specific client diagnosed with social isolation is:

Level	Hours per week at senior center
1	None
2	1–2
3	3–5
4	6–7
5	8

Levels are assessed at the start and end of a study period, with the difference between the two levels representing the goal-attainment score.

Nursing process intervention follows. A major component of interventions, in addition to those relevant to each specific nursing diagnosis, is the use of a self-concept enhancing protocol with all clients. This protocol consists of a synthesis of concepts and principles of older adult nursing care and Carpenito's format for nursing diagnosis (Carpenito, 1987). Protocol focuses on therapeutic communication and activities related to each of the parts of self-concept. We have developed, and continue work on "Imperatives in Therapeutic Communication with Older Adults." Currently, we identify these as:

Respect	Touch
Attend	Support
Listen	Care
Assist	Understand

In the self-concept enhancing activities section of the protocol each self-concept component and related activities for nursing intervention emphasis are included:

Self-concept component	Activities to promote
Self-esteem	Social functions, classes
Role performance	Family, friend interactions; recreational, vocational pursuits
Personal identity	Group and individual study regarding ethnicity, age, and spiritual self
Body image	Exercises, grooming, imagery

For evaluation, we note the client's general appearance and behavior, as well as how they report their mood, activity, and self-care. Progress in goal attainment is looked at in regular post-conferences and periodic case reports. Faculty regularly audit charts of each client in their case loads. A pilot study of goal attainment has been done and is ongoing. The goal of this study is to document concurrent application of the self-concept protocol and client goal attainment. Seven clients, 6 female and 1 male, with a mean age of 69 (57–88) were studied. Five live alone and 2 live with 1 or 2 others; there is an average of 1.4 group social activities per week. All 7 do their own cooking, 3 drive automobiles, and there was an average of 5 clinic visits per client during the 7-week study period. Sixteen nursing diagnoses were studied including nutrition, anxiety, activity intolerance, and grief. The study revealed an improvement of at least 1 goal attainment level in 12 of the 16 diagnoses, or 75 percent.

Enjoyment, the second element of synergy in the nurse subsystem, is experienced in getting to know and understand clients and appreciating the wide variety of healthy aging processes; it is also found in seeing clients make healthy changes and achieve goals. The third element, enthusiasm, is reflected in our efforts to deal effectively with administrative, management, and client-care challenges, and it, in turn, enhances our efforts. Our efforts will expand this fall when we start another site in a primarily Hispanic west downtown area. Most students demonstrate enthusiasm frequently by returning for additional elective credit hours when they are offered at the clinic.

A task force of project staff and professional advisory board members has just begun work on plans for permanent funding.

ENVIRONMENT

Having considered the nurse subsystem, I now refer to the human environment, the Highland Center staff and volunteers. Energy is provided in their cheerful tolerance of our takeover every Friday afternoon and in valuable services, such as music and food for our parties, client transportation, and photography of our activities. Enjoyment is experienced in the exchange of information relating to health topics and client-care resources. Enthusiasm is most apparent in referrals and when volunteers enroll as clients themselves.

CLIENT

Having considered the nurse and the environmental subsystems, I turn now to the client. Energy here comes from making self-care changes and in relating the benefits to other center members, who then often also become GEHM clients. Enjoyment is experienced in receiving attentive and appropriate care. They often express appreciation of the stimulation provided by the young students. Enthusiasm is demonstrated in return visits and in referrals of family members and friends for individual services as well as health seminars and support groups.

EFFECTS

The elements of energy, enjoyment, and enthusiasm interact among the nurse, the client, and the human environment in a synergistic manner to render ongoing order from our lively chaos. On a deeper level, participation in the GEHM clinic system helps meet the developmental needs for intimacy, generativity, and integrity of young, middle-aged, and older adult nurses, clients, and center staff.

REFERENCES

Carpenito, L. J. (1987). *Nursing diagnosis, application to clinical practice.* Philadelphia: J.B. Lippincott.

Carter Center. (1988). Atlanta, Emory University.

Folstein, M.F., et al., (1975). Mini mental state: A practical method of grading the cognitive state of the patient for the physician. *Journal of Psychiatric Review, 17,* 189.

Lawton, M.P., Moss, M., Fulcomer, M., & Kleban, M.M. (1982). A research and service oriented multilevel assessment inventory. *Journal of Gerontology, 37,* 91–99.

Mangen, D.G., & Peterson, M.A. (1982). *Research instruments in social gerontology.* Minneapolis: University of Minnesota Press.

Orem, D. E. (1985). *Nursing, concepts of practice.* New York: McGraw-Hill.

Schultz, P.R. (1979). *Primary health care to the elderly.* Denver: Medical Care and Research Foundation.

Yesavage, J.A., Brink, T.L., Rose, T.L., et al. (1983). Development and validation of a geriatric depression rating scale: A preliminary report. *Journal of Psychiatric Research, 17.*

12

Home Health Care through an Academic Nurse-Managed Center

Esther L. Acree, MSN, SpClNsg, FNP
Veda J. Gregory, MSN, SpClNsg, FNP

Health care in the United States has come full circle in the twentieth century, from home care settings to institutional care settings and back to home health care (Hogstel, 1985). Several factors contribute to this trend toward home care: (1) demographic changes, (2) pressure by the public and private sector to contain health care cost, (3) advances in medical technology for home care, (4) an overall interest in providing care in a more accessible environment, and (5) an increasing focus on wellness, prevention, and health maintenance.

The demographic changes show nearly 12 percent of the U.S. population is over the age of 65 and this number is increasing yearly (Halamandaris, 1985). Furthermore, this older population is expected to have doubled between 1980 and the year 2000 (Johnson, 1985). Ramage (1985) recognized that this group has more instances of chronic illness and social isolation than other age groups. Today's society has become so mobile that the support of an expanded family is obsolete. Halamandaris (1985) goes on to state that as the mortality rate reduces there will be a direct increase in disability and therefore a greater need for home care and long-term care.

In addition to the fact that there is no national health policy on home health care, Medicare and Medicaid programs have not been cost-effective, nor have they provided the optimum benefits to the people needing health care: Medicare provides no preventative services for older adults and Medicaid is available only to a minority of the poor. These health care programs pay for limited parts of the home care package and then only if the individual or family meets certain criteria for eligibility, such as a hospital stay or care ordered by a physician (Spiegel, 1983). Implementation of the Diagnostic Related Grouping (DRG) based payments (Coleman and Smith, 1984) has been one mechanism to contain health care cost. DRGs have affected various client aggregates and caused an increased need for home health care services. These aggregates are the aged, the chronically ill, the handicapped, the high-risk mother and infant, and the client discharged from the hospital with limited support systems.

According to Spiegel (1983) most people want to be an active partner in making decisions that directly affect their lives. The concept of home care allows the individual to play a central role in his or her health care. People feel that home care offers more control over what happens and do not feel as helpless as they may in a hospital setting. Consumers of all ages are taking a partnership role in their personal health and medical care through an interest in self-care and informed decision making. Many consumers advocate a comprehensive model of health service delivery. There are currently limited resources available for these services (Hogstel, 1985).

An ideal home care model includes health promotion, disease prevention, and health maintenance. Traditional home health care agencies spend a great deal of time caring for more acutely ill clients and limit the provision of health promotion, illness prevention, and health maintenance services to the population in need. These changes have ethical implications for nurses providing home care and for the institutions. The dilemma involves cost-effectiveness and quality care, and how to provide both. Nurses, having a key role in community-based care, should support diversified and innovative models for providing comprehensive home health care. A creative approach to the delivery of this type of home health care is within the concept of a nurse-managed center.

Schools of nursing seek to create nursing centers, or academic nurse-managed centers, as they are presently called (Barger, 1986). These centers are based in schools of nursing and directed by faculty, staff, and students. Academic nurse-managed centers in the United States have similar critical issues that are currently being researched.

Clientele is a major issue. Clients frequently have one common feature: they are either inadvertently forgotten, or they are underserved by the traditional health care system (Barger, 1986). The underserved and forgotten groups receiving health care through nursing centers include the elderly, mothers and children, the disabled, the poor, and the homeless. Ultimately, these centers strive for client diversification to maintain the integrity of nursing care and to prevent a two-tiered system.

A second issue is the determination of services to be offered. In a recent survey, Barger (1986) found that services frequently offered by nurse-managed centers include health assessment, chronic and common acute illness management, health education and counseling, and referral and collaboration with other agencies. Most academic nurse-managed centers continue to receive primary support from their college or university, which allows long-term care to be provided when necessary (Barger, 1986). However, the economic viability of academic nursing centers is an issue to be examined in light of services, student clinical experiences, faculty practice, and research.

Personnel issues in academic nurse-managed centers involve students and faculty. Barger (1986) points out that the manner in which administrators address the needs and requirements of the staff will determine the effectiveness and longevity of these programs. If faculty practice and student learning experiences are recognized, the various areas of expertise will ensure high-quality care. The issue of staff coverage during the summer months has been resolved in several centers by allowing faculty members who have nine-month academic contracts summer employment with the agency, and by incorporating service in the center as part of twelve-month appointments (Herman and Krall, 1984). These academic nurse-managed centers have numerous faculty with the needed specialty skills.

HOME HEALTH CARE THROUGH AN ACADEMIC NURSE-MANAGED CENTER MODEL

Philosophy

The philosophy of Indiana State University (ISU) provides for a mission statement that challenges each school to meet its purpose of education, research, and human service endeavors. The goals developed by the school of nursing's nurse-managed center (NMC) seek to develop programs that contribute to health promotion, illness prevention, rehabilitation, and health maintenance of individuals and families. The NMC is committed to providing direct health service programs in addition to providing educational experiences for students. Therefore, the Sycamore Nursing Center (SNC) and the faculty of the junior-year community health nursing course deem it most appropriate to its mission to develop an innovative program of home health care within its NMC.

History

The purpose for developing the home health program through the SNC at the school of nursing was to provide clinical educational experiences focusing on health maintenance and illness prevention in the home setting. The services were provided primarily to clients and their families in a five-county geographical area.

The goals of the home health program were twofold: (1) to provide clinical experiences for junior and senior nursing students in the community health nursing and leadership courses, and (2) to provide home health care services to clients and families discharged early from other home health agencies or not qualified for such services due to cost containment regulations of Medicare and Medicaid.

The home health care program began working with the local Visiting Nurses' Association (VNA) in the summer of 1985. A referral mechanism was developed between the two agencies to provide for continuity of care for clients and their families. During the summer two faculty and one junior student (who was completing a nursing elective in community health nursing) visited 6 families referred from the VNA. The caseload has now grown to over 60 families being visited by 10 community health students as part of their clinical experience. Currently, 4 senior community health students have developed charts, criteria for visits, discharge criteria, audit forms, and marketing strategies as a year-long project in collaboration with faculty.

Utilization

The focus of this home health program is health promotion, illness prevention, and health maintenance of clients with stable chronic health problems. Services include nursing care ranging from short-term to long-term maintenance care, health education, referrals, and collaboration with other health care providers. Clients are selected primarily through referrals from the local VNA. Clients and their families are persons who must be discharged from the VNA service because of third-party reimbursement regulations and who have been assessed by the visiting nurses as needing further health maintenance and illness prevention. Approximately 60 percent of the clients are older adults who have one or more chronic illnesses, and who typically live alone or with a spouse, but rarely with other family members. The home health care program also accepts referrals from the following community agencies: Family Service Association; school corporations; Women, Infant, and Children Supplemental Nutrition Program; county health departments; local hospitals; Child and Adolescent Services; older adult programs; and selected private physicians.

Elements for Effective Operation

Numerous elements were found to be necessary for effective functioning of home health care through the SNC. These elements include a physician advisor, operational policy, marketing mechanism, year-round personnel, and community and colleague support.

The physician, who is also the county health officer, functions largely in an advisory capacity providing guidance in developing policy and protocol, and medical consultation as needed.

Legal policies were developed in cooperation with the university lawyer to satisfy faculty concern about the legal issues involved in operating a home health care program. All nursing students and faculty are covered by the university liability insurance during clinical experiences. Home health care is provided by students only during regular clinical times and only by faculty who have a contract with the university. All clients and their families contract with the home health program and give written consent for home visits and provided care. Family health records are kept on all clients seen by faculty and students.

Marketing activities were not emphasized the first year of operation due primarily to the fear of inadequate staffing for semester breaks and summer vacations. During the 1986–87 academic year, four senior community health nursing students developed a brochure listing the services offered by the SNC. These brochures were distributed throughout the community prior to May 31, 1987. The director and coordinator of the SNC are in the process of contacting all area physicians and community agencies to explain the scope of the home health care services and elicit feedback regarding concerns. The physicians and agencies who have already referred to the home health program are satisfied with the services. This satisfaction has been expressed in writing, by phone, and through feedback from clients and their families. A slide/tape and video presentation promoting the home health care services is also being developed.

Personnel for the home health program for the 1986–87 academic year consisted of 2 faculty who are family nurse practitioners, 10 junior nursing students, and 4 senior community health nursing students. The problem of summer coverage for 1987 was resolved by the ISU administration who provided a summer stipend for the two faculty positions. There is a continuing effort to promote faculty practice within the SNC. The SNC at ISU has both the community and colleague support necessary for survival of a NMC.

Problems Encountered

Providing a home health program through the SNC has been a tremendously exciting and rewarding adventure. However, it has presented a few problems. The first problem is the need for a structured advisory board whose members represent faculty and appropriate community people. Currently, the center is functioning under the advisement of a faculty nursing council and the community advisory board of the entire school of nursing. This is inappropriate because the needs of the SNC are different from those of the school of nursing. The second problem has been staffing adequate faculty during summer months. With the increase in referrals related to the marketing strategies, the question is whether two faculty positions in the summer will be adequate in the future. The third and last problem is the need for a master plan for evaluation of outcomes and total program evaluation.

Future Plans

In regard to the establishment of a financial base, the SNC has elected not to participate in third-party reimbursement at this time. There has been discussion of the benefits of charging a nominal fee for services, and the ISU business office has been asked to recommend an appropriate nominal fee.

Future plans of the SNC include the addition of high-risk prenatal, postpartum, and newborn assessments through referrals from local hospitals and the Maternal Health Clinic; substance abuse assessment and referral in the home; and the care of the chronically mentally ill in the home.

It is anticipated that students from the Community Health Nursing Master's Program at ISU will also use the SNC for research projects and clinical learning experiences.

Even though the SNC has tools for rating client and student satisfaction, as well as a preliminary tool for auditing, these tools still need to be tested for reliability and validity.

IMPLICATIONS FOR COMMUNITY HEALTH NURSING

The challenge currently facing the health care industry is how to provide for quality, yet cost-effective health care. Community-based care must be offered through coordinated efforts so that a variety of needs can be met. The local VNA has asked the director of the SNC to participate on a task force to address the care needs of the community's indigent in the home health arena.

The Community Nursing and Ambulatory Care Act is becoming a reality. It would seem that the provision of community nursing centers would provide for more autonomous and less physician-oriented care in a more economical, efficient manner. However, nursing needs to develop health care policy in the area of innovative nursing models so that community-based nursing centers and academic nurse-managed centers can provide both on-site and home health care programs. There must be continual evaluation of the cost-effectiveness and the quality of nursing's standards of care. It is now necessary for the concept of home health care to be reexamined as a vital component in the health promotion, acute treatment, and long-term maintenance of the aged, handicapped, ill, and other high-risk populations.

Academic nurse-managed centers and traditional home health care agencies should network and collaborate to provide quality care to clients during this time of changing trends and economic shifts in health care. The next 20 years will challenge academic nurse-managed centers involved in providing home health care to follow in the footsteps of Lillian Wald—with new agency configuration, new roles, and new challenges in home care services.

REFERENCES

Barger, S.E. (1986). Academic nurse-managed centers: Issues of implementation. *Family and Community Health, 9*(1), 12–22.

Coleman, J.R., & Smith, A. (1984). DRG's and the growth of home health care. *Nursing Economics, 2* (6), 391–395.

Halamandaris, V.J. (1985). The future of home care. *Caring, 5*(10), 4–11.

Herman, C.M., & Krall, K. (1984). University sponsored home care agency as a clinical site. *Image: The Journal of Nursing Scholarship, 16*(3), 71–75.

Hogstel, M.O. (1985). *Home nursing care for the elderly.* Bowie, MD: Brady Communications Company, Inc.

Johnson, K.A. (1985). Exploring home health care opportunities as a result of the prospective payment system. *Caring, 5*(4), 54–60.

Ramage, N.B. (1985). In-home health care services: A policy perspective. *Family and Community Health, 8*(2), 11–21.

Spiegel, A.D. (1983). *Home health care.* Owings Mills, MD: National Health Publishing.

13

Encouraging One-Hundred Percent Faculty Participation in an Academic Nursing Center Practice Plan

Norman D. Brown, EdD, MS, RN

It takes full faculty cooperation, communication, and commitment to operate three neighborhood clinics that provide basic health services for over 500 individual clients annually. For three years, the Wellness Center Project (WCP), an academic nursing center supported by the Division of Nursing at the University of Texas at Tyler, has provided primary health care for senior citizens, abused adolescents, and women who have entered their third trimester of pregnancy with no prior prenatal care. Throughout its years of operation, nursing faculty and students have provided over 10,000 client contacts for the individuals in the Wellness Center Project caseload. All clinical services are provided by nursing faculty in cooperation with a variety of health and human services providers. The evolution of this nurse-managed clinic system has required at least five years of concerted effort by the participating nursing faculty and was greatly facilitated by the academic campus setting where the University of Texas educational program is based.

Historically, university-based nurse educators have enjoyed a profound freedom from non-nurses whose influence in the design and content of nursing curriculum has been oppressive in the hospital setting (Carter, 1987). The evolution of academic nursing centers is a critically important step in the development of nursing education because of the autonomy they afford nursing educators in implementing their own curricula and clinical expectations in an open environment (Carter, 1987). The freedom to develop unique learning experiences for both faculty and students has been a key element in the development of the WCP. The faculty members of the University of Texas at Tyler believe that the movement toward academic nursing centers presents an opportunity for nursing education to evolve to a higher level of organization. However, at UT Tyler, as at most other schools of nursing, there is no universal agreement regarding the direction in which faculty practice, and therefore academic nursing centers should move (Millonig, 1986). In order to provide each faculty member with a voice in the operation of the WCP, a management scheme has been developed that matches each faculty member's talent and time with a direct role in the operation of the WCP.

FORMALIZING THE WELLNESS CENTERS PROJECT: A MANAGEMENT PLAN

The following is an overview of the management plan that represents the current administrative practices of the WCP. Each level of responsibility requires incremental increases in commitment of a faculty member's time and talents. Each level of participation is described and followed by a brief description of the incentives realized by faculty members who choose to participate at that level. In general, the faculty member's responsibilities to the WCP increase as they progress through the system from level one to level three. All faculty members are expected to participate in the management scheme and are rewarded according to their level of commitment. The willingness to participate actively in the WCP activities is considered a desirable characteristic of all potential faculty members.

Level One. Level one participation is expected of all full-time faculty members regardless of rank or tenure status. This level of commitment simply requires active participation of the WCP Advisory Committee. This commitment calls for attendance at the quarterly meeting of this group and provides each faculty member with the opportunity to offer advice and consent regarding the direction of the WCP clinical services.

Incentives for participation include: (1) tenure and promotion credit for professional development and community service opportunities, and (2) opportunities to explore ideas and options for the development of the WCP clinical services.

Level Two. Participation at this level indicates a desire to assume a leadership role in the WCP and participation at this level of responsibility is optional for each full-time faculty member. WCP leadership roles include any of the following: (1) chairing a special interest subcommittee, (2) developing research related to the clinical services provided, and (3) acquiring contracts for clinical services.

Incentives for participation at this level are the same as level one *plus* the following: (1) research development opportunities, as evidenced by the development of preproposals, (2) potential for salary enhancement, and (3) enhanced professional development, such as opportunities for consultation and active participation in research.

Level Three. This level represents the administrative positions of the WCP and the greatest commitment of a faculty member's time and talents. At this level a faculty member may hold the title of Project Director, Principal Investigator, or Clinical Site Manager.

The project director is responsible for the overall operation and periodic evaluation of the WCP. This includes conducting the quarterly advisory committee meetings, communicating the purpose of the WCP to all interested parties, and exploring ways to enhance the WCP through grants, contracts, and other creative avenues.

Principal investigators are individuals who have developed research projects that utilize the resources of the WCP. These individuals have generated research designs that can be conducted in one of the clinical sites operated under the WCP. The research design has been reviewed and approved by the advisory committee members, and the responsibility for the conduct of the research rests with this individual.

Clinical site managers are the faculty members who take responsibility for the direct supervision of clinical services delivered by the WCP. These individuals will deliver services, supervise volunteers and other clinic personnel, see that clinical areas are maintained, and assure that all records are compiled in a professional manner. These individuals communicate regularly with the project director and prepare quarterly and annual reports regarding their particular clinical service.

Incentives for the third level of participation include those noted for the level one and level two *plus* the following: (1) salary enhancement, and (2) consideration for release time.

The premise upon which this management plan is based acknowledges that collegial involvement in all aspects of the WCP is an essential element for both the continued success of this project and the evolution of the profession of nursing. The concept of professional evolution and the broadening of the role of the nurse educator from a clinical and classroom setting to a position of independent practice is repleat with questions and conflicts. The definition of faculty practice, how should it be rewarded, and whether all nurse educators should be involved in academic nursing center practice are questions many educators believe constitute the heart of the practice issue (Tornay, 1987). The management plan outlined is one attempt to resolve in

a professional manner the questions and conflicts surrounding faculty practice.

The faculty members at UT Tyler believe that nursing is a force that can
bring great benefits to society through the provision of extremely cost-
effective health services. The WCP management plan allows for the growth
and development of additional clinical services in concert with the professional development and interests of each faculty member. In its current form,
the WCP successfully provides both faculty and students with opportunities
to practice their clinical skills, conduct research, and provide meaningful
community service. Future success will be fostered through the active
participation of these faculty members in the planning, implementation, and
evaluation of clinical services described in this management plan.

REFERENCES

Carter, M.A. (1987). Professional practice: Those who can't practice—Teach.
  Journal of Professional Nursing, 3, 131.

Millonig, V.L. (1986). Faculty practice: A view of its development, benefits,
  and barriers. *Journal of Professional Nursing, 3*, 166–171.

Tornay, R. (1987). Toward faculty practice. *Journal of Nursing Education, 1*,
  137.

14

Addressing the Health Needs of Congregations: Who Are the Nurses in Churches?

Mary Ann McDermott, EdD, RN

Nursing's roots lie with the deacons and deaconesses, monks and nuns of earlier centuries, in their commitment to the Church, and demonstrated in their care for the sick and the poor. The idea of lay professional nurses as ministers of health within a church congregation, however, is relatively new. Limited references to this new role were evidenced in a review of the literature ("Nurse's notebook," 1983; Westberg, 1986; "Parish nurses," 1987; Striepe & King, 1987; Striepe, 1987; Westberg & McNamara, 1987), and a data base that describes the characteristics of nurses in churches of various denominations has been developed. The data make it apparent that nurses in this new role are "blessed" with a variety of gifts that make them uniquely attractive to church congregations striving toward holistic health. I have been able to infer twelve beatitudes from the data that I believe have application to nurses in other nurse-managed centers as well.

Data were collected through a questionnaire distributed to nurses practicing in such positions who were attending the Granger Westberg Annual

The author acknowledges the assistance of Erin Mullins, BSN, RN, who assisted in analyzing the Parish Nurse Survey data. The Granger Westberg Annual Symposium on Parish Nursing referred to in the article was held September 25, 1987 at Lutheran General Hospital, Park Ridge, Illinois. The Parish Nurse Resource Center is funded by the Lutheran General Health Care System, Congregational Health Partnership Project, Parkside Center, 1875 Dempster St., Park Ridge, Illinois 60068, Ann Solari-Twadell, Director.

Symposium on Parish Nursing in September 1987 in Park Ridge, Illinois. A total of 37 questionnaires, primarily from the midwest, were returned. An accurate count of the number of nurses practicing in a church/parish setting is not available, however the recently established Parish Nurse Resource Center estimates there are approximately 50 programs in operation and an additional 30 being developed.

DEMOGRAPHIC DATA

Nurses who responded to the survey generally had a great deal of inpatient experience prior to assuming their current position of "Parish nurse" or "Minister of health." The nurses were almost exclusively female; there was only one male respondent. Of the 37 nurses surveyed, 26 were 40 years of age or older, and all had been married; 2 of the nurses were widows and 2 had been divorced. Seventeen of the nurses reported holding a baccalaureate degree in nursing or some other field, and 9 of these nurses reported also holding a master's degree in nursing or some other field. All of the nurses reported previous nursing experience ranging from 5 or less years to over 20 years, with 33 nurses reporting previous hospital inpatient employment. Almost all the nurses queried had been previously active as volunteers in some type of church work. Follow the educational preparation with a rich and varied work and life experience record and you have the beatitude: Blessed be the parish nurse for she has had a generalist education and previous employment that have resulted in a broad variety of skills.

Queried as to the denomination of the congregation served, Lutheran parishes were identified by 17 of the respondents. Other denominational sponsorships included Roman Catholic, Methodist, and Presbyterian. Thirty-one of the 37 nurses identified themselves as members of the denomination they served; 22 nurses were serving in their own congregations. It is conceivable that nurses such as those just described permeate just about every church congregation in this country. As the largest group of health care professionals in this country, our sheer numbers lend a credibility to the beatitude: Blessed be the parish nurse for she is available and accessible to most congregations.

Are these parish nurses practicing as volunteers? Or, if salaried, from what source is their salary derived? Only two parish nurses reported full-time salaried positions. Twenty-seven of the respondents hold part-time (20 hours or less) salaried positions. Twelve of the nurses reported volunteer status or a combination of volunteer and salaried status. The primary salary source in most instances is a combination of sponsorship by a hospital and the congregation. Only 6 nurses reported the congregation as the sole salary provider. Twenty-five of the parish nurses are currently employed elsewhere, and the greatest number of these (11) work in the hospital inpatient setting. It seems that the part-time (20 hours or less) position would be an ideal role for a faculty practice role. In any instance, what a bargain: Blessed be the parish nurse for she is cost-effective.

PARISH NURSE RESPONSIBILITIES

Parish nurse responsibilities reported were comprehensive, both in services rendered and age groups served. The dominant service responsibilities included health counseling, health teaching, and referral. Health screening and volunteer training were reported as secondary service responsibilities. Less frequently mentioned were hands-on care; home, hospital, and nursing home visitation; and the facilitation of support groups. Adults, 30 years of age and older, are the parishioners most often served by the nurse. Preschool and school-age children are also frequently served in school settings. Parish nurses reported less involvement with adolescents and with mothers and infants than with the other age groups. Familiarity with the resources available in a particular community was mentioned repeatedly as a mandate for the parish nurse role. Respondents reported that having at least a rudimentary background in community health nursing, previous involvement in hospital discharge planning, and ongoing working relationships with personnel from agency resources, was critical to their support of individuals and families. Blessed be the parish nurse for she is knowledgable about community resources and the process of referral.

Nurses in general have learned the art of juggling—tossing and catching, keeping both employees and clients satisfied at the same time, and making it all look easy—better than other health care workers. Parish nurses reported a considerable amount of juggling in their new roles and all but two of the respondents were the first persons to occupy the position within their congregation. They have learned to juggle personnel, time, conflicting needs of systems, providers, and patients. What a balancing act! Rather than labeling her a juggler, I have chosen more sophisticated terminology: Blessed be the parish nurse for she has a high tolerance for ambiguity.

Parish nurses reported that they transformed and redefined the skills utilized in the crisis orientation of their inpatient setting experience to prioritize in their new positions. Several parish nurses commented that they knew how to distinguish the chronic crisis that needs monitoring from those events that are more acutely urgent. Blessed be the parish nurse for she focuses on priorities and she may even reorder the priorities if assessment data change.

The nurses were asked to recall two or three primary factors that influenced their decision to assume their current position in parish nursing. A strong person-orientation with a focus on empowerment of parishioners and process was evidenced in most of the responses. However, like nurses in general, parish nurses have been less than enthusiastic about quantitative hard outcome data. "Doer" rather than "evaluator" seems to be a term that more accurately characterizes the parish nurse role. All areas of evaluation—self, peer, consumer, employer, and process and program outcome—appeared limited. The beatitude, however, is positive: Blessed be the parish nurse for she is process oriented.

PERSONAL CHARACTERISTICS OF THE PARISH NURSE

Caring is an intangible entity, a happy mixture of many gifts and virtues. Asked to identify personal and professional characteristics most important to their success as parish nurses, words such as *love, kindness, empathy, trustworthiness, hospitality*, and *graciousness* were used to describe the selfless caring that these nurses demonstrate. From their responses you might infer that they are pushovers for a worthy cause—several even acknowledged that maybe they care too much. The respondents often referred to their work as a "vocation" or "calling" and used quasi-religious terms of "gift" and "grace." Caring was also described in terms of interpersonal communication that focused on listening skills as well as enabling, facilitating, and promoting skills. Blessed be the parish nurse for she is caring.

Parish nurses were articulate in expressing their dissatisfaction with unrealistic expectations of work performance in the time allotted. Expectations were viewed as potential causes of guilt, stress, and burnout. One respondent, salaried at 20 hours, wrote: "It is impossible to restrict the time. I would like to be present for 40 hours (or more) without feeling I am being 'unfaithful' to the stated goals, expectations, etc. I feel if I'm ever salaried for 40 hours I'll have a real problem explaining why I'm not doubling what I'm now doing!"

Benefits from personal satisfaction however, outweighed the frustrations. The opportunity to establish long-term trusting relationships within the worshipping community, with both the parishioners and colleagues on the parish staff, and the opportunity to follow through with a holistic nursing care approach over extended periods of time were mentioned repeatedly. The opportunity to influence change was evident in phrases such as "making a difference" and "seeing the impact." Satisfaction was well described by one nurse who wrote ". . . being *everything* that I am and being able to bring out my full potential as a nurse." Blessed be the parish nurse for she possesses generosity of spirit, both of time and talent. And, blessed be the parish nurse for she is committed, dependable, and persevering.

Are nurses who currently practice in the parish role pioneering a new role in nursing? I mentioned that all but two of the respondents were the first in their congregations to be in this innovative role; many nurses identified frustrations associated with the newness of the concept: role definition, role boundaries, and role expectation. Nevertheless, most of the respondents described the role as challenging and exciting. Recall that nursing has a heritage and tradition in and of the church. Perhaps a parish is not so much innovative in placing a nurse on the parish team, as just long overdue. Each nurse who chooses or is chosen for parish nursing will be a pioneer simply because the role will be new to that nurse and to most congregations. However, the parish nurse is urged to look over her shoulder occasionally, remembering and thanking Fabiola, Marcella, Helena, and Placilla, to name just a few who have journeyed before. Blessed be the parish nurse for she has a heritage and tradition of pioneering.

Parish nurses by their own admission value a strong personal faith, an enthusiastic and joyous approach to life, and view nursing as a ministry. Acknowledgment of God's direction in the decision process in assuming the parish nurse role was also evidenced. Blessed be the parish nurse for she is a believer . . . in God, in clients, in nursing, in herself, and in a better world, here and in the hereafter.

SUMMARY AND IMPLICATIONS

The Lutheran Church in the Midwest is taking leadership in advancing the role of nurses providing holistic health care to congregations of different denominations. The survey reported here provides a data base that hopefully will stimulate interest in parish nursing and encourage other studies of the parish nurse as a community health provider. It is interesting to note that this role has developed over the past few years concurrently with the concept of nurse-managed centers, also having its roots in the Midwest. The deep commitment of the parish nurses recorded in this study has the potential for creating vulnerability in these individuals. The documentation of activities and outcomes that may validate a full-time position is critical in preventing stress, guilt, and subsequent burnout. Additional rationale for documentation includes program development, historical tracking, and tracking communication across settings.

The data support the necessity of matching opportunity with life-style. The older, experienced, married nurse is able to combine her established interest and activity in church community life with her professional talents in the parish nurse role.

Because of the nature of the position, nurses are usually the sole health provider on the parish team. Coupled with limited participation in professional organization activities, the need for ongoing, self-initiated continuing education, and the establishment of professional networking is viewed as necessary to the prevention of isolation and stagnation. The minimum of a baccalaureate nursing education appears most appropriate for the parish nurse functioning as an autonomous generalist in community health, caring for a specific population. As with other new nursing roles, the ultimate success of the parish nurse role is highly dependent on the implementation of formal, regular evaluation. Evaluation should be of both the program and the individual's performance, encouraging and facilitating growth, appropriate change, and affirming the nurse in this new and challenging role.

REFERENCES

Nurse's notebook. (1983). *Nursing 83, 13*(1), 82.

Parish nurses meet spiritual needs in Chicago. (1987). *American Nurse, 19* (5), 1.

Striepe, J. (1987). *Parish nurse manual II: Curriculum.* Sioux City, IA: Iowa Lakes Area Agency on Aging.

Striepe, J., & King, J. (1987). *Parish nurse manual I.* Sioux City, IA: Iowa Lakes Area Agency on Aging.

Westberg, G. (1986). The role of congregations in preventative medicine. *Journal of Religion and Health, 25*(3), 193–197.

Westberg, G., & McNamara, J. (1987). *The parish nurse: How to start a parish nurse program in your church.* Park Ridge, IL: Parish Nurse Resource Center.

15

Academic Nursing Centers: An Assessment after a Decade

Sara E. Barger, DPA, RN, FAAN
William C. Bridges, Jr., PhD

The concept of an academic nursing center, a place which Lang described as a "model teaching center for students, where the best of nursing practice could be observed, learned, and tested" (Lang, 1983), originated in the early 1970s when several schools of nursing opened nursing centers. A report of such a center from the Adelphi University School of Nursing and Molloy College Department of Nursing appeared in the literature in 1973 (Jones, Pagel, & Wittman, 1973). Montana State University's School of Nursing at Bozeman described a similar model in 1977 (Hauf, 1977). By the early 1980s, the professional journals contained many descriptions of these centers which seemed to be appearing in all regions of the country (Riesch, Felder, & Stander, 1980; Ossler et al., 1982; Cobb, Kerr, & Pieper, 1980; Mezey & Chiamulera, 1980; Arlton & Miercort, 1980; Grimes & Stamps, 1980).

This literature presents a high degree of consensus as to the purpose of these centers. Four purposes that are cited consistently include providing:

1. An educational experience for students
2. A practice site for faculty
3. A setting for faculty and students to conduct research
4. Nursing services to the community (Lang, 1983; Riesch, Felder, & Stander, 1980; Ossler et al., 1982; Cobb, Kerr, & Pieper, 1980; Mezey & Chiamulera, 1980; Jones, Pagel, & Wittman, 1973; Williamson, 1980; Aydelotte et al., 1987; Barger, 1985; Boettcher, 1985a; McEvoy &

Vezina, 1986; Baird & Benner, 1985; Thibodeau & Hawkins, 1987; Duffy & Halloran, 1986)

While these purposes were cited often, any assessment of these centers' success in accomplishing their purposes was noticeably absent. Since academic centers have been in existence for at least a decade, it is now appropriate for such an assessment. First, an overview of a descriptive study on academic nursing centers will be presented. Next, the development of an assessment system will be described. This system can be used by centers to determine if they are meeting their objectives. The system was applied to the existing data base of academic nursing centers and the results of that pilot study are presented. Finally, the findings are discussed, including implications for the future of academic nursing centers.

DESCRIPTIVE STUDY OF NURSING CENTERS

In 1987, the authors completed a preliminary study to gather demographic data and to establish a data base on existing academic nursing centers. Data were organized around center demographics and the four purposes of faculty practice, student education, community service, and research (Barger & Bridges, in press). A survey instrument was sent to 68 schools that earlier studies had identified as operating a nursing center (Barger, 1986; Boettcher, 1985b). Of the 66 schools that responded (97%), 45 (68%) indicated that they had a nursing center. Data provided by these 45 schools established the initial data base of academic nursing centers.

Center Demographics

Nursing centers participating in the study included older, well-established centers, as well as newer ones. Centers ranged in age from 1 to 12 years in existence, with a mean age of 5.8 years and a standard deviation of 2.8 years. The college/school-of-nursing building was the most frequent location (38%) cited, followed by the senior citizens center or building (24%). Twenty-four percent of the centers had two sites. Generally these centers served the community, but 27% of these served only senior citizens. Some centers served only the homeless, the university community, or low-income populations.

Although schools typically had several sources of support for their centers, the schools themselves were paying about half the cost. Client fees and third-party reimbursement covered 15% of the budget while contracts, consultations, and in-kind support covered another 15%. On an average, federal grants were supporting about 8% of these budgets, and other grants 9%.

Center Purposes

When respondents listed their own centers' purposes, 89% included community service, 61% listed student education, 48% listed research, and 43% listed faculty practice. Included in the data collection were specific data for each purpose.

Faculty Practice. The average size of the faculty in schools with nursing centers was 33 with 6 faculty members (18%) participating in the center in the previous year. The majority (67%) of respondents indicated that practice in the center was negotiated as part of the workload with no additional reimbursement received. Only 13% indicated the option of a faculty-practice plan with additional reimbursement.

Student Education. Findings on student education indicated that an average of two courses used the center for clinical experience. One of these courses was at the senior level, the other at the masters level. However, a mean of only 25% of seniors and 6% of masters students had experience in the center. A mean of 0% of doctoral students had experience in the center.

Research and Scholarship. Centers averaged one student and three faculty research projects conducted in the center since opening. There was a mean of one research and one nonresearch manuscript submitted for publication per center with a mean acceptance rate of 100% for both types of manuscript.

Service. Service data were collected on age groups served, services provided, and hours of operation. A breakdown of the client population by age group indicated that the largest percentage of the total client population was in the 65-and-over age group but that the standard deviation was also large. The next largest age group served was the 18–34 group. A smaller percent of the client population included children; 12% were under age six and 7% were 6–17. While 89% of the centers provided services to senior citizens, only half provided any services to children and adolescents.

Respondents indicated that a wide range of services were available through their nursing centers. Physical assessment was provided in 93% of the centers, screening in 82%, health risk assessment in 80%, counseling in 77%, health education groups in 69%, home health services in 38%, and psychotherapy in 18% of all centers.

The hours of operation of these centers varied widely. Three centers offering midwife delivery or home health services were on call 24 hours a day throughout the year. All other centers were open an average of 25 hours a week during the academic year, 9 hours a week during school holidays, and 19 hours a week during the summer.

The findings of this descriptive study indicated varying degrees of commitment to and accomplishment of the four purposes of faculty practice, student education, community service, and research that are reported with such consistency in the literature. In addition to providing a beginning data base on academic nursing centers, the findings inspired the authors to propose the development of a scale or assessment system that could be used by centers to measure success in fulfilling each purpose area.

DEVELOPMENT OF THE ASSESSMENT SYSTEM

The first step in developing an assessment system was to combine all the components of each purpose into a score that would reflect a center's commitment to a purpose. To accomplish this, an equation was formulated that added all the components together. Some components were expressed as ratios or fractions, while others were multiplied by coefficients or weights. The refinements to the equations were made so that the score would more accurately reflect the center's commitment to the purpose. These refinements were somewhat subjective, based on the authors' knowledge of nursing centers, and therefore had a large influence on the final score. These equations were then used to score each purpose.

Faculty Practice Score. The two versions of the equation for determining the faculty practice score are shown in Figures 1 and 2. Since these centers are usually community based, the first formula (Figure 1) was weighted toward a higher expectation of community health faculty participation. Similarly, if the center served only senior citizens, extra weight was divided equally between faculty prepared in community health and those prepared in gerontology (Figure 2). Both equations were formulated in such a way that proportions of faculty were used instead of total faculty in order to avoid bias in favor of larger schools.

$$F = 4 \left(\frac{A}{B}\right) + \frac{C}{D}$$

When

F = Faculty practice score
and
A = Community health faculty in center
B = Community health faculty in school
C = All other faculty in center
D = All other faculty in school

Figure 1
Faculty Practice Score Equation for All Centers
Except the Sites Serving Only Senior Citizens

$$F = 2 \left(\frac{A}{B}\right) + \frac{C}{D} + 2 \left(\frac{E}{F}\right)$$

When

  F = Faculty practice score
    and
  A = Community health faculty in center
  B = Community health faculty in school
  C = All faculty in center other than community health and geron-
    tology faculty
  D = All faculty in school other than community health and geron-
    tology faculty
  E = Gerontology faculty in center
  F = Gerontology faculty in school

Figure 2
Faculty Practice Score Equation for Centers Where
Primary or Secondary Site Serves Only Senior Citizens

A separate equation was formulated for centers serving only senior citizens because of the large percentage (27%) of centers serving only this population. However, the same logic could apply to other specialized centers serving other population groups, for example pregnant women, children, and so on. Additional equations were not formulated for these centers because there were not as many of them.

Student Experience Score.   The student experience equation considered two variables: the total number of courses offered at all levels using the center for student experience, and the proportion of students at each level (junior, senior, masters, and doctoral) who received experience in the center (Figure 3). Again, the equation was formulated to use proportions to avoid bias in favor of larger schools. However, schools with masters and doctoral programs did have a slight advantage since they could add up to two points if 100% of these students received experience in the center. In spite of this advantage, it was not expected that the scores of these schools would be higher because descriptive statistics had revealed so little participation by masters and doctoral students.

Research and Scholarship Score.   This equation required the considera- tion and weighting of many factors. The total number of studies in the center per faculty member per year was important. This proportion considered the total number of faculty in the school, even if they did not participate in the center. The second fraction in the equation considered manuscripts, research and nonresearch, both accepted for publication and unpublished. The

$$X = A + B + C + D + \frac{E}{F} + \frac{G}{H} + \frac{I}{J} + \frac{K}{L}$$

When

X = Student experience score
and
A = Number of junior-level courses using the center
B = Number of senior-level courses using the center
C = Number of masters-level courses using the center
D = Number of doctoral-level courses using the center
E = Number of junior students with experience in the center
F = Total number of junior students
G = Number of senior students with experience in the center
H = Total number of senior students
I = Number of masters students with experience in the center
J = Total number of masters students
K = Number of doctoral students with experience in the center
L = Total number of doctoral students

Figure 3
Student Experience Score Equation

greatest weight was given to a published research manuscript; less but equal weight was given to a published nonresearch manuscript and an unpublished research manuscript; and the least weight was given to an unpublished nonresearch manuscript. It should be noted that all of these types of scholarship received credit. The proportion was determined on the basis of manuscripts per faculty working in the center per year. The resulting total equation is shown in Figure 4.

Service Score. The service score considered access to services for populations in all age groups. Range or diversity of services was also included in the equation. Finally, availability was measured by the proportion of the total hours in a week (168) that a center was open during the academic year, summers, and holidays. Figure 5 presents the procedure for determining the service score.

Total Score. In order to determine a center's aggregate performance in all four purpose areas, the authors decided to calculate a total score. This score was the sum of the individual scores for the four purposes.

Determination of Scores' Ranges and Minimums

After the equations for all purposes were formulated, the range of possible scores was determined. Then a minimum acceptable score was set for each

$$R = \frac{A}{B} + C + [(\frac{4D + 2E + 2F + G}{B}) + H]$$

When

    R = Research & scholarship score
       and

    A = Total number of studies in the center
    B = Age of the center
    C = Total number of faculty in the school
    D = Number of published research manuscripts resulting from the center
    E = Number of published nonresearch manuscripts resulting from the center
    F = Number of unpublished research manuscripts resulting from the center
    G = Number of unpublished nonresearch manuscripts resulting from the center
    H = Number of faculty in the center

Figure 4
Research and Scholarship Score Equation

$$S = A + B + (\frac{C + D + E}{168})$$

When

    S = Service score
       and

    A = 1 point for each age group served up to a maximum of 8 points.
    B = 1 point for each type of service up to a maximum of 11 points.
    C = Center's hours per week during academic year
    D = Center's hours per week during holidays
    E = Center's hours per week during summer

Figure 5
Service Score Equation

purpose (Table 1). This minimum was the lowest score a center could receive and still meet a minimum performance standard (set by the authors) for that purpose. The methodologies for determining these minimum scores are discussed in the following sections.

Faculty Practice Score.   If all of the faculty in the school participated in the center, the highest possible score was 5. In centers other than those serving only senior citizens, the minimum passing score was set at 2, based on 50% of the community health faculty participating but no other faculty participating. In centers serving only senior citizens, the minimum acceptable score was also 2, based on 50% of the community health faculty and 50% of the gerontology faculty participating but no other faculty participating.

Student Experience Score.   Although the authors realized that it was possible for the student experience scores to be higher, they decided that the highest possible student experience score would be set at 12. Realistically, it is unlikely that more than two courses per level (junior, senior, masters, and doctoral) would use the center for experience for 100% of the students at each level. A minimum acceptable score was set at 4. This score was based on all schools having a baccalaureate program but not necessarily a masters or doctoral program. Therefore, the minimum was one course at both the junior and senior level, with all students at each level having an educational experience in the center.

Research and Scholarship Score.   Again, the scoring potential was large here. However, a maximum score of 7 was calculated on the basis of all faculty in the school conducting one study per year in the center and having one research and one nonresearch manuscript published. Certainly it would be possible for faculty to be more productive than this "maximum" score. A

Table 1

Scoring System for Service Components

Component	Highest Possible Score	Lowest Passing Score
Access for all age groups	8	2
Range of services	11	3
Availability		
Academic year	1	.23
Holidays	1	.23
Summer	1	.23
Total availability	3	.69

minimum passing score was set at 2.1. This score was based on 10% of the faculty participating, each conducting one research study per year in the center. Also included in the minimum was one unpublished research manuscript or two unpublished nonresearch manuscripts per faculty member participating in the center per year. Thus, it was only required that manuscripts be written, not that they be published, since some faculty members might feel publication to be beyond their control.

Service Score. The highest possible score was in the area of service (Table 1). It was possible to obtain 8 points for access by serving all age groups and 11 points for range of services by providing all types of services. Availability was measured by determining the proportion of the total hours in a week that services were available during the academic year, holidays, and summers. For example, centers open 40 hours a week out of the total hours in a week of 168 during the academic year, holidays, and summers, would have a total availability score of 0.71, or 0.23 each for the academic year, holidays, and summers. If a center had 24 hour-a-day service availability during the academic year, holidays, and summers, the availability score would be 3. Thus, the total maximum service score was calculated to be 22. A minimum passing score was set at 5.69. This minimum was based on a center providing at least three services to two age groups 40 hours per week during the academic year, summers, and holidays.

Total Score. The highest possible score was determined by adding the maximum scores in the four purpose categories and was found to be 46. The lowest passing total score was calculated in the same manner and found to be 13.79. As Table 2 indicates, highest possible scores ranged from 22 to 5 for the different purposes, while minimal passing scores in these same areas ranged from 5.69 to 2.

After the equations were formulated and possible ranges and minimum passing scores determined, the authors applied the assessment system to the existing data base of academic nursing centers. The SAS computer software

Table 2
Scoring System for Nursing Center Purposes

Purpose	Highest Possible Score	Lowest Passing Score
Faculty practice	5	2
Student experience	12	4
Research and scholarship	7	2.1
Service	22	5.69
Total Score	46	13.79

package was used to perform the calculations. Scores were calculated for each school, for each purpose area, and a total score was determined. Descriptive statistics were then calculated for these scores.

APPLYING THE ASSESSMENT SYSTEM

Descriptive statistics are presented in Table 3. In the area of faculty practice where the highest possible score was 5 and the lowest passing score was 2, scores ranged from 0 to 4.75. The mean was 1.39, the median 1.0, and the standard deviation was 1.25.

For student experience, where the highest possible score was 12 and the lowest passing score 4, the scores ranged from 0 to 10.13. The mean was 2.86, the median 2.18, and the standard deviation 1.96. Thus, although some schools had high student experience scores, most fell on the lower end of the range.

Research and scholarship scores ranged from 0 to 2.04. The mean was 0.18, the median 0.02, and the standard deviation 0.36. Here, the highest possible score was 7 and the lowest passing score was 2.1. Data show scores on the lower end of the range with little dispersion.

Service scores, both in possible scores and in actual scores, were the highest of all the purposes. The highest possible score was 22 and the lowest passing score was 5.69. The actual scores ranged from 3.04 to 18.71. The mean was 11.84, the median 11.18, and the standard deviation was 3.70.

In addition, the authors' realization that the service score was a composite of three very distinct and different measures—access for all age groups, range of services, and availability—moved them to conduct an in-depth analysis of the service purpose (Table 4). For the measure of access, with a maximum

Table 3
Descriptive Statistics for Scores of Nursing Centers for Each Purpose

Purpose	Range	Mean	Median	Standard Deviation
Faculty practice	0–4.75	1.39	1.00	1.25
Student experience	0–10.13	2.86	2.18	1.96
Research and scholarship	0–2.04	0.18	0.02	0.36
Service	3.04–18.71	11.84	11.18	3.70
Total Score	6.40–29.80	16.06	14.81	5.08

Table 4
Descriptive Statistics for Components of Service Score

Component	Range	Mean	Median	Standard Deviation
Access for all age groups	2–8	3.13	2.50	3.00
Range of services	1–11	6.62	7.00	2.04
Availability				
Academic Year	0–1	0.21	0.15	0.24
Holidays	0–1	0.12	0.00	0.27
Summers	0–1	0.18	0.10	0.25
Total Availability	0–3	0.50	0.24	0.75

possible score of 8 when all age groups were served, scores ranged from 2 to 8. The mean was 3.13, the median 2.5, and the standard deviation was 3.0. Range of services could and did vary from 1 to 11. The mean was 6.62, the median 7.0 and the standard deviation 2.04.

Availability was highest during the academic year, with a mean of 0.21, a median of 0.15 and a standard deviation of 0.24. Next were summers with a mean of 0.18. The time service that was least available was holidays, with a mean of 0.12. Total availability scores were rather poor, with a mean of 0.5, indicating that services generally were available much less frequently than 40 hours per week throughout the year.

When the centers' service scores were examined, their best performance lay in range of services offered and the poorest performance lay in availability (Table 5). Ten centers received passing scores for all service measures. Thirty-one centers passed all measures except availability. One center passed range of services and availability and one center passed only access.

Total scores, which were additions of the scores from each purpose, ranged from 6.4 to 29.8. The mean was 16.06, the range 14.81, and the standard deviation was 5.08.

Next, data were analyzed to determine the number and percentage of centers with passing scores for each purpose (Table 6). The highest pass rate was for service. Forty-three centers (95.5%) passed in this area. Passing rates were much lower for faculty practice and student experience, 28.2% and 22.2% respectively. The poorest passing rate was 0% in the area of research and scholarship.

The final part of the analysis examined the ability of centers to balance success in all purpose areas. As Table 7 indicates, no centers received passing scores for all purposes. Two centers received passing scores in three areas; faculty practice, student experience, and service; but not in research. Six

Table 5
Number of Centers with Passing Scores and Failing Scores by Service Component

Number of Centers	Access All ages	Range of Services	Availability
10	+	+	+
31	+	+	−
1	−	+	+
1	+	−	−
2	Missing data in at least 1 component		

+ = Passing score
− = Failing score

Table 6
Number and Percentage of Centers with Passing Scores by Purpose

	Number of Centers with Passing Scores	Percentage of Centers with Passing Scores
Faculty practice (N = 39)	11	28.2
Student experience (N = 45)	10	22.2
Research and scholarship (N = 40)	0	0
Service (N = 45)	43	95.5
Total (N = 45)	27	60.0

centers received passing scores in student experience and service, but not in faculty practice and research. Eight centers had passing faculty practice and service scores, but failed research and student experience. Seventeen schools succeeded in only one area, service. Two schools received no passing marks. Ten schools had missing data required to perform the calculations and so a score could not be calculated for at least one purpose.

Table 7
Number of Centers with Passing Scores and Failing Scores by Purpose

Number of Centers	Faculty Practice	Student Experience	Research and Scholarship	Service
0	+	+	+	+
2	+	+	−	+
6	−	+	−	+
8	+	−	−	+
17	−	−	−	+
2	−	−	−	−
10	Missing data in at least 1 purpose area			

+ = Passing score
− = Failing score

DISCUSSION

The assessment system developed by the authors and applied to the existing data base identified both strengths and weaknesses in existing academic nursing centers. Centers were most successful in meeting their service purpose, although availability was a problem. This finding is not surprising considering that 89% of all respondents stated in the original survey that service was one of their center's purposes. This result is also in keeping with the service focus of the profession.

However, the assessment system identified a large disparity between desirable scores and actual scores in both the areas of faculty practice and student experience. Less than 25% of the centers had passing student experience scores, even though 61% of the respondents said that student education was one of their centers' purposes. Less than one-third of all centers had passing faculty practice scores, which is not surprising given that only 43% of the respondents listed faculty practice as a purpose.

In the area of research, 48% of all respondents listed research as one of their center's purposes, although no center had a passing score in research. In considering possible reasons for this finding, one must also question if the centers' research scores are indicative of low research productivity within the profession, or if faculty who conduct research in other sites are more productive than those faculty providing service in nursing centers.

An examination of how well centers balanced their purposes revealed difficulty in this area. The majority of centers were meeting only the service mission and nothing more. If they continue to meet only this purpose, the authors believe that these centers will probably cease to function, for there are certainly others who can provide these services at lower cost than those in the academic environment. Instead, the authors believe that nursing-center entrepreneurs were on the right track in the early 1970s when they included faculty practice, student experience, and research in the mission statements of their centers. It is true, perhaps, that they did not know then the obstacles they would face in the process of implementation. Nevertheless, these purposes are lofty and worthy of the struggle.

This assessment system and its application are only first efforts and in need of further refinement. The results presented here must be viewed more as a demonstration of the assessment system than as a definitive evaluation of the performance of nursing centers. The authors acknowledge that these findings are a function of their scoring of the existing data supplied by the centers. Nevertheless, whether center directors use the system presented here or another system, it is important that those involved in nursing centers begin to evaluate what they are doing, because, to paraphrase noted management expert Peter Drucker, success can only be measured in terms of what one is trying to accomplish (Drucker, 1973).

REFERENCES

Arlton, D., & Miercort, O. (1980). The challenge for student learning opportunities. *Journal of Nursing Education, 19*(1), 53–58.

Aydelotte, M.K., et al., (1987). *The nursing center: Concept and design,* Kansas City, MO: American Nurses' Association.

Baird, S.C., & Benner, R. (1985). Keeping a university well with a health promotion clinic. *Nursing and Health Care, 6*(2), 107–109.

Barger, S.E. (1985) Evaluating a nurse-managed center. *Nurse Educator, 10*(4), 36–39.

Barger, S.E. (1986). Academic nursing centers: A demographic profile. *Journal of Professional Nursing, 2*(4), 246–251.

Barger, S.E. & Bridges, W. (in press). An assessment of academic nursing centers. *Nurse Educator.* (Mar–April 1990).

Boettcher, J.H. (1985a). *Nursing centers in academia and faculty job satisfaction.* Unpublished doctoral dissertation, the University of Texas, Austin.

Boettcher, J.H. (1985b, May 11). Personal communication.

Cobb, A.K., Kerr, M.A., & Pieper, B. (1980). Nurse managed clinics: An approach to graduate community health nursing education. *Image, 12*(2), 34–36.

Drucker, P. (1973). Managing the public service institution. *Public Interest, 33*, 43–60.

Duffy, D., & Halloran, M.C. (1986). Meeting the challenge of multiple academic roles through a nursing center practice mode. *Journal of Nursing Education, 2*, 55–58.

Grimes, D., & Stamps, C. (1980). Meeting the health care needs of older adults through a community nursing center. *Nursing Administration Quarterly, 4*(3), 31–40.

Hauf, B. (1977). An evaluative study of a nursing center for community health nursing student experiences. *Journal of Nursing Education, 16*(8), 7–11.

Jones, A., Pagel, I., & Wittman, M.E. (1973). Nursing center for family health services. *Journal of the New York State Nurses' Association, 4(1),* 33.

Lang, N. (1983). Nurse-managed centers. Will they thrive? *American Journal of Nursing, 83*(9), 1291.

McEvoy, M.D., & Vezina, M. (1986). The development of a nursing center on a college campus: Implications for the curriculum. *Journal of Advanced Nursing, 11*, 295–301.

Mezey, M., & Chiamulera, D. (1980). Implementation of a campus nursing and health information center in the baccalaureate curriculum. Part I: Overview of the center. *Journal of Nursing Education, 19*(5), 7–10.

Ossler, C.C., Goodwin, M.E., Mariana, M., et al., (1982). Establishment of a nursing clinic for faculty and student clinical practice. *Nursing Outlook, 30*(7) 402–405.

Riesch, S., Felder, E., & Stander, C. (1980). Nursing centers can promote health for individuals, families and communities. *Nursing Administrations Quarterly, 4*(3), 3–4.

Thibodeau, J.A., & Hawkins, J. (1987). Evolution of a nursing center. *Journal of Ambulatory Care Management, 10*(3), 30–39.

Williamson, J. (1980). Faculty practice in a nursing center: An integrated model. In *Interpreting and implementing faculty practice roles in nursing education.* (p. 17). New York: National League for Nursing.

16

Nurse-Managed Centers: The Future Of Health Care Delivery (Purpose and Uses)

Richard J. Fehring, DNSc, RN

When you hear or read about the shortage of nurses in the United States you usually associate it with a shortage of nurses who maintain on-site hospital and acute medical services. This shortage is real, important, and a great problem. But, there is another type of nurse shortage in this country that is just as real and perhaps more important to the future of nursing and health care: this is the shortage of professional nurses who meet the variety of present and emerging health problems in this country—problems such as health care for the homeless, care of the elderly who are sick and well, care for people with chronic health problems, health promotion and disease prevention, development of a wellness life style, teenage pregnancy, family planning, well-baby and well-child care, to name a few. These problems fit well into nursing practice and nursing models of health and as such are the type of health problems encountered in nursing centers.

Nurse-managed centers could be the vehicle for nurses to take a stronger leadership role in meeting the major health needs in our country, and also could be a way of attracting more people into the nursing profession. Some reasons for this are that nursing centers free professional nurses to practice nursing; they allow people direct access to nursing services; they allow nurses to take primary responsibility for health problems; and the length and nature of the relationship with the client is not dictated by another profession. Nurse-managed centers offer avenues for nurses to take the lead in and become experts for our present and future health problems.

At the beginning of the twentieth century there was a young woman who dropped out of medical school because she realized that nursing was the profession in which she could best meet the health needs of the poor in New York City. This nurse, and another nurse friend, started the first nursing center in this country. Their nursing center became a model for other nursing centers and many of the nursing leaders in our country at that time had professional experience in this center. Their center eventually became the catalyst for what we call "public or community health nursing"; it was also the vehicle for national legislation on health care for children, and was the site at which "modern" nursing was developed. This nursing center was called the Henry Street Settlement and the nurse who started it was Lillian Wald (Wald, 1902). If nursing continued to develop in the model of practice that Wald demonstrated, nursing and health care would be much different today.

This article presents examples of modern-day Lillian Wald's and modern day Henry Street Settlements (nursing centers), and the purposes and uses for today's nursing centers. In addition, examples of other historical nursing centers will also be given because we need to realize the many foundations of our profession and find stimulation in the examples of these nursing pioneers.

PURPOSE AND USE

There are essentially four purposes for nursing centers discussed in the literature: (1) to provide service to the community; (2) to provide sites for professional nursing practice; (3) to provide settings for the education of students; and (4) to provide sites for nursing research. These purposes are not unique and could be applied to hospital-based or community-based nursing, but there is a qualitative difference that is not readily apparent. This presentation describes those differences, first by examining some of the uses of and services provided in nursing centers, and then the nature of the practice, education, and research that is done in nursing centers.

Present-day nursing centers are used in a variety of ways to meet the health needs of people. One of the most urgent and most publicized health problems of our country are the health needs of homeless people. These problems are essentially nursing problems. Nurses have attempted to meet the needs of homeless people long before publicity and money were available. The needs of the homeless are often provided for through a nursing center or clinic. For example, the Pine Street Clinic, located in a shelter for homeless in Boston, has been providing health care since the mid-1970s. In 1985, nurses who wrote an article on the clinic reported that they saw 110–120 men nightly in the clinic, which is open every night of the week (Lenehen, McInnis,

O'Donnell, & Hennessey, 1985). At the Third National Conference on Nurse-Managed Centers, Dr. Jo Ellen Murata presented the UCLA School of Nursing Clinic for the Homeless, situated in the Union Rescue Mission shelter in Los Angeles. In 1985 they had 9,675 primary-care clinic visits and provided experience for 51 students. Besides primary care they also provide food, clothing, showers, delousing, and rehabilitation programs. At the Fourth National Conference on Nursing Centers in May 1988 the Community Kitchen Health Clinic was presented. This clinic is operated in conjunction with the Community Soup Kitchen in Lexington, Kentucky and the University of Kentucky School of Nursing. Another example is St. Benedict's Health Care Clinic for the homeless. This clinic was started in 1980 and operates as a collaboration between St. Benedict's Parish Meal Program and St. Mary's Hospital in Milwaukee, Wisconsin. The clinic has an outreach clinic at the meal site, which is open two nights a week, and a clinic with formal office hours in the parish rectory. The clinic's coordinator is a masters-prepared nurse who coordinates a team consisting of a primary-care physician, a social worker, and a psychiatrist. Services include health assessments, screenings, immunizations, health classes, street outreach, health counseling, referral, advocacy, and mechanisms for volunteer work and socialization for the homeless client. The clinic also serves as a site for student practice both graduate and undergraduate students from Marquette University. The St. Benedict's clinic and the UCLA clinic receive funds from the Robert Wood Johnson and Pew Memorial Foundations.

In addition to the homeless, many nursing centers are sites for health care to indigent populations. An example of such a nursing clinic/center is the nursing clinic in the Langston Dwelling housing project in Washington, DC (Ossler, Goodwin, Mariani, & Gillis, 1982). This nursing clinic was developed by the faculty to serve as a practice site for undergraduate nursing students in community health at Catholic University of America. Another example is the Marquette University Nursing Center with outreach clinics in various low-income housing projects and sites where the Hmong and Laotian populations live.

The health needs of the sick and well elderly is another emergent and existing health issue in the United States. The problems of the elderly include helping the elderly stay healthy, as well as helping them cope with chronic health problems. The vast majority of elderly are not coping with their health problems and maintaining a wellness lifestyle in the hospital or nursing-home setting. There are a number of nursing centers and clinics that provide services for the elderly that have been reported in the literature or at conferences. Neufield and Hobbs are two faculty members from the University of Saskatchewan that staff a nursing clinic for the elderly in a senior highrise; the school of nursing at the State University of New York has a nursing clinic in a senior center in Brooklyn; the Pacific Lutheran College of Nursing has a nursing clinic for elderly in the Highland Senior Center; and the University of Indiana School of Nursing has a nurse practitioner wellness clinic for older adults. Services in these nursing centers include health education, counseling, various health screenings, exercise groups, weight-loss services, stress management, home visits, and reminiscence therapy, among others. The University of Texas Nursing Center nurses provide health fairs for the elderly at various sites where elderly live or gather. Both the Pacific Lutheran and the University of Saskatchewan centers are based on Orems' self-care model. In the future, masters-and/or doctorally-prepared clinical specialists and nurse practitioners will be providing nursing care in many of the elderly housing projects and apartment complexes throughout the country.

Many of the academic nursing centers provide health and wellness services to the faculty, staff, and students of various campus communities. Examples include the Health Place Nursing Center at the University of Wisconsin at Oshkosh, and the Wellness Center at Alverno College. Pace University School of Nursing has a clinical practice units (CPU) for primary health care that is situated in an old college infirmary. The nursing center is based on the Neuman Systems Model. This CPU calls to mind another historical nursing center: the Loeb Center, developed in the late 1950s by Lydia Hall. Lydia Hall called the Loeb Center a "center for nursing" and saw the nurse as the chief therapeutic agent in this center. The University of Florida School of Nursing provides a family health clinic for residents of family housing on the university campus, and Lehman College in New York has a campus health clinic that provides women's health services.

Another unique setting for a nursing clinic or center is the church or synagogue. Because nursing is of a wholistic nature, the church, which is already providing spiritual care, is a natural setting for nursing. The church often has rooms available, it is a common gathering place for people, and the church's pastor often is in contact with and knows many of the health needs of a congregation. In the late 1970s and early 1980s, Granger Westberg, a Lutheran minister, advocated and developed a number of wholistic health clinics in church settings. The clients would come to these clinics and be seen by a physician, minister, and nurse. He learned, however, that these clinics were too expensive to operate and provide primary medical care. He is now advocating and developing the concept of a parish nurse or a nurse as a "health minister" in the church setting. A book is available on the parish nurse or how to start a parish-nurse clinic (Westberg & McNamara, 1987). The Iowa Lutheran Hospital has a certification program for parish nurses. Nurses who have completed their parish nurse certification program are now managing and staffing small church-based nursing clinics. Marquette University has two church-based clinics and Loyola University of Chicago School of Nursing faculty and students provide home health care services through a parish in Chicago.

These preceding examples are just a few of the types and uses of nursing clinics/centers in the United States. There are many other models, settings, and uses, including women's health clinics, family planning clinics, stress management clinics, school-based clinics, and neighborhood clinics. In the future there will be many other models of health care delivery in which nursing centers will be the primary source of innovation. These innovative models of health care delivery and services will be needed in order to meet the changing health patterns in the United States and to meet the health problems of a modern society.

PRACTICE, EDUCATION, AND RESEARCH

A unique aspect of nursing and health is that a lasting change in health behaviors often occurs only through a trusting relationship with another person. When Lillian Wald began her nursing center she decided that she did not want to use the missionary approach and dictate health care to the people, but rather to live within the neighborhood and effect change through a trusting relationship. Nurses who work with the homeless, especially the mentally ill and substance abusers, know that change occurs only through a trusting relationship, and then only after a long period of time. Nursing centers provide professional nurses with a practice site at which such relationships can develop and where the nurse has control over practice and the length of the relationship. Nursing centers are also often located in places where people gather (senior centers, meal sites, shelters, churches) so that they are convenient to the client, less threatening, and are not to be mistaken for medical clinics. A nursing center should be a pleasant place to be for the nurse and the client alike. Lillian Wald had women's clubs at her nursing centers, often organized community picnics, and developed safe play areas for children (Wald, 1902).

The key to practice in the nursing center is that nurses have control. This control means that they have direct access to clients, are able to dictate the length of time the client needs to be in a therapeutic relationship, that the primary model of practice for the center is health and nursing, and that the nurse has the freedom to be innovative in the type of care given and with the type of interventions and evaluation methods utilized. For example, if a nurse wants to teach a client a relaxation technique or recommend a low-fat diet, or teach a jogger proper stretching exercises, the nurse would not have to go through the physician. Another issue is that the nurse has the primary responsibility for the health care of the client, or as Lydia Hall stated, the nurse is the "chief therapeutic agent" (Hall, 1963). As such, the nurse provides the locus of care and the other health professions are auxiliary care providers. The nurse in the nursing center is not there to facilitate the practice of another health profession. Nurses who work in the nursing center setting soon find that there is more to nursing than the taking of medical orders and vital signs, watching monitors, transporting patients to other health professions, and admitting and discharging patients. Furthermore, nurses who have not worked in such settings are often afraid because they do not know how to practice in an independent manner. A nurse in a nursing center is forced to develop a repertoire of interventions, assessments, referral sources, and consultants.

Because nursing is the focus and control of health care in nursing centers, nursing centers make ideal sites for student learning. Many of the freestanding nursing centers and all of the academic nursing centers provide sites for student learning and faculty practice. A common practice in nursing schools is to have 4–10 students occupy a hospital unit. The faculty member in charge comes to the unit the day before the students arrive and assigns patients to the students. This practice of education, however, has a lot of deficits and abuses. In the hospital it is the physician, and not the nurse, who is the chief therapeutic agent and the professional who is emulated. Students are often assigned to watch physicians carry out medical procedures. In the hospital setting, students often must follow a population not on that unit. How many times do students take courses in child or adolescent nursing and end up taking care of an elderly patient, or how often do you find four students and staff members assigned to the care of one patient? Not the well elderly, the adult person coping with chronic health problems, the teenager, children, the new mother, in fact not many people at all, are coping with their health problems in the hospital setting.

In the hospital the faculty and students maintain guest status and do not have direct responsibility for nursing care. Often students and faculty are in the way, and because hospital services are designed to facilitate a medical model of health, patients are discharged with very short stays and often with need of health education and nursing care. Finally, in the hospital setting the focus of care is often on techniques, for example, how to start IVs, administer injections, or interpret monitors. This reinforces students' thinking that they are not practicing nursing unless they are carrying out techniques. This "technique mentality" is not altered until they have practiced in a hospital for a year or so, and can be a source of boredom for the professional nurse.

In contrast, the nurse in a nursing center is the chief therapeutic agent and nursing faculty often carry a practice and become role models for, or colleagues with, the students. The faculty and students in nursing centers are not considered "guests," and the nursing centers are based on nursing models of health promotion. The length of the therapeutic relationship with a client in a nursing center is directed by the nurse. Populations such as the well elderly and teenagers come to these clinics because they are provided services in their own settings. To illustrate, if you want to work with adolescents, an ideal place would be to have a nursing clinic in a high school. A housing project for the elderly would be an ideal site for a wellness clinic for older adults.

The research and innovations that have and can come about through nursing centers are endless. Because nursing centers are nursing-focused and the nurse who practices in a nursing center has control over practice, the setting fosters research and innovations. The development of public and community-health nursing through Wald's nursing centers, the innovative treatments and practice that Sr. Kinney developed in her nursing clinics for polio victims, and the forerunners of the Planned Parenthood clinics for women developed by Margaret Sanger are just a few examples of historically innovative nursing centers. Today there is potential for many more. Research in today's nursing centers is minimal, largely because much of the nurses' energy is focused on the development and maintenance of the clinics. There has been a variety of research conducted through nursing centers, including studies on health behaviors, compliance, health promotion, cost effectiveness, quality assurance, marketing, and the role of the independent practitioner. About 55–70 percent of nursing centers have research as a goal; very few, however, actually have specific role functions for research or support research service. Likewise, there are not many doctorally-prepared nurses who are conducting research in nursing centers. In the future, nursing centers will become more likely places for research and development. Doctoral programs in nursing will be linked with nursing centers and nursing centers will be the laboratory for doctoral student research. Furthermore, research in nursing centers will increase because, as Susan Riesch, DNSc, RN, FAAN stated at the Third Conference on Nurse-Managed Centers in April 1986, practice in nursing centers attracts a "bright, creative group of nurses."

CONCLUSION

In 1978, at the annual American Public Health Association convention, Dr. O. Marie Henry presented a paper on demonstration centers for nursing practice and called for the development of nursing centers in a variety of settings (Henry, 1978). She predicted that such nursing centers would result in a significant improvement in the nursing care rendered to patients. Ten years later many of our nursing centers are still struggling and developing and are not the 24-hour-a-day, 7-day-a-week centers that Dr. Henry envisioned. In fact, the centers more closely resemble the picture that accompanied an AJN article by Lang, the keynote speaker at the Second National Conference on Nursing Centers (Lang, 1983). This picture shows numerous small buildings (nursing centers) as flowers in a garden that are just budding in their development. The picture also shows a nurse watering the buildings as a symbol of nourishment. If nursing centers are ever to be the 24-hour-a-day, 7-day-a-week centers Dr. Henry envisioned, and are ever to make an impact on our nation's health are provision, then nursing will have to make a bigger commitment to these centers and realize that the professional nurse will be able to meet the future needs of health only by being free to have control of practice and free to pursue health problems where they occur.

REFERENCES

Hall, L.E. (1963). A center for nursing. *Nursing Outlook*, November, 805–806.

Henry, O.M. (1978). *Demonstration centers for nursing practice, education, and research.* Presentation to the Association of Graduate Faculty of Public Health and Community Health Nursing, annual meeting of the American Public Health Association, Los Angeles.

Lang, N.M. (1983). Nurse-managed centers: Will they survive? *American Journal of Nursing, 83* (9), 1290–1293.

Lenehan, G.P., McInnis, B.N., O'Donnell, D.O., & Hennessey, M. (1985). A nurses' clinic for the homeless. *American Journal of Nursing, 85*(11), 1236–1240.

Ossler, C.C., Goodwin, M.E., Mariani, M., & Gillis, C.L. (1982). Establishment of a nursing clinic for faculty and student clinical practice. *Nursing Outlook, 20*(4), 402–405.

Wald, L.D. (1902). The nurses' settlement in New York. *American Journal of Nursing, 2*(8), 567–574.

Westberg, G.E., & McNamara, J. (1987). *The parish nurse: How to start a parish nurse program in your church.* Park Ridge, IL: Parish Nurse Resource Center.